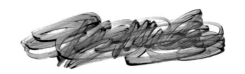

D1558375

SMILING
THROUGH TEARS

Other Upton Books Publications

Confabulations:
Creating False Memories, Destroying Families
by Eleanor Goldstein with Kevin Farmer, 1992

True Stories of False Memories
by Eleanor Goldstein and Kevin Farmer, 1993

Beware the Talking Cure:
Psychotherapy May Be Hazardous to Your Mental Health
by Terence W. Campbell, Ph.D., 1994

Survivor Psychology:
The Dark Side of a Mental Health Mission
by Susan Smith, 1995

Psychology Astray:
Fallacies in Studies of "Repressed Memory"
and Childhood Trauma
by Harrison G. Pope, Jr., M.D., 1997

SMILING THROUGH TEARS

By Pamela Freyd
and Eleanor Goldstein

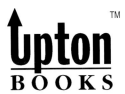
Upton™
BOOKS

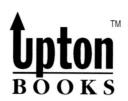

Upton ™

BOOKS

A division of

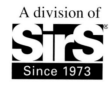

Since 1973

Social Issues Resources Series, Inc.
P.O. Box 2348
Boca Raton, FL 33427

Library of Congress Cataloging-in-Publication Data

Freyd, Pamela.
    Smiling through tears / by Pamela Freyd and Eleanor Goldstein.
       p.   cm.
    Includes bibliographical references and index.
    ISBN 0-89777-125-7
    1. False memory syndrome. 2. False memory syndrome—Humor.
I. Goldstein, Eleanor C. II. Title.
RC455.2.F35F73 1997
616.85'822390651—dc21

                                         97-13345
                                           CIP

The cartoons were selected by the authors to
reflect the themes of the various chapters. It in no
way signifies that the cartoonists endorse the
ideas or thoughts portrayed in this book.

Linda Manis, Managing Editor
Michelle McCulloch, Book Design
Kathryn Piercey, Permissions

Tens of thousands of families have been torn asunder by false accusations that have emerged from regression therapy. Adult children have come to believe they were abused by parents they once loved and respected. It appears that they have acquired false memories.

Cartoonists have captured some of the major ideas behind the movements that created the milieu in which false memories thrive. With a few strokes of the pen and a few words, they have cut to the heart of the matter. They make us smile even in the face of great tragedy.

We hope to enlighten the general public about the abuses taking place in our society because science and justice are being abandoned in the face of hysteria and illogic. We also hope that after reading this book, which includes about 125 cartoons, afflicted families will come to understand that this social phenomenom has reached public consciousness. With awareness, solutions will be forthcoming.

We know that many families are still separated because of this false belief system. We hope that the humorous aspects of this book will enable them to smile through their tears.

Pamela Freyd
Eleanor Goldstein

Critical Reviews

"*Smiling Through Tears* is an amazing book, at once both thoroughly informative and devastatingly witty. It is a thorough and highly readable analysis of all issues surrounding the "recovered memory" hysteria that has battered the North American family scene. Cogently described is the rise, thanks to the ratings-chasing talk shows and Bradshaw-esque family-hating psychgurus, of a vacuous psychobabble as the dominant interpretive discourse facilitating America's reconstruction as psychic disorders solve all the problems humans encounter in life. It is just a coincidence, of course, that these newly perceived psychic disorders require therapeutic intervention, available, as it happens, at a not inconsiderable cost, from those who have engineered this transformation, the new therapeutic industry. Also described are the terrible witchhunt trials that have resulted as this intellectual illness infected the courtrooms of our judicial system, carried on in there in the persons of bogus, scientifically illiterate "expert" witnesses, to waste resources and ruin lives. But it does all this accompanied by some of the funniest cartoons you will ever read.

The book is a primer on all the relevant issues: the science of memory, hypnosis, multiple personality disorder, post-traumatic stress disorder, satanic ritual abuse, pop psychologies and even the relevant legal precedents. These and more are all discussed in writing that is easily understandable but sacrifices nothing by way of scientific validity. And hilarious cartoons from the *New Yorker*, Dilbert and Doonesbury, among others, add laughter and entertainment along the way, while reinforcing the points made in memorable fashion.

Other recent books have covered some of the same ground, but in hundreds more pages and thousands more syllables. Scientific research, sociological realities, psychological findings, and psychiatric concepts have never been easier to understand. Calvin and Hobbes explain victimhood in a way that says it all.

Maybe the death knell for the recovered memory quackery was Gary Ramona's successful suit against his daughter's therapist. Maybe it was the appellate reversal of George Franklin's criminal conviction. After reading this book I'm convinced it was when the brilliant cartoonists represented here felt that tug on the compass of their wit that pointed them in the direction of this century's greatest episode of psychic foolishness, so that a curative ridicule could start to be applied.

Those that would benefit the most from this wonderful book—the recovered memory fanatics—generally being a self-righteous, humorless lot, probably won't read it. Everyone else—lawyers, judges, parents, experts, doctors, psychiatrists, counsellors, etc.—should. There will never be a more comprehensive or readable exposition of this entire topic for anyone who has to grapple with the issues in their personal or professional life, or anyone just interested. Tragically, the issues covered affect nearly everybody today, and understanding them and what is happening will never be easier than by reading this book.

You'll learn and understand, and amidst the learning, you'll laugh with this marvelous book."

**—Alan Gold,
Criminal Defense Attorney, Toronto, Canada**

"The psychologists, psychiatrists and all of the variously credentialed "therapists" who pollute thinking by spewing out misinformation about vulnerability, memory, abuse and trauma, and peddling their absurd notion of a healing process that involves "wallowing in pain" and "pointing the finger of blame" are good fodder for cartoonists. This art form, more swiftly and effectively than words alone could ever do, strips away the arrogant professional facades, demonstrating that "the clothes have no emperor."

Smiling Through Tears is a powerful book for several reasons: First, it brings together a priceless collection of images that serve to cut down to size the pathetically ignorant charlatans who are profiting from interfering in personal lives, damaging families, contaminating justice and distorting common sense.

Second, it provides accurate, concise and clearly expressed information about "therapy gone crazy" and summarizes key points from the solid research which is being used to effectively challenge the principles and practices of this entirely unsubstantiated but effectively marketed nonsense.

Third, it places the idea of repressed memory into the broader social context of a moral panic where this phenomenon most assuredly belongs; and it summarizes most eloquently the recent history of the rise and fall of one of this century's most hideous intrusions.

And finally, without making false promises, it gives hope and encouragement to those who are trying to deal with the devastating effects of repressed memory therapy on their own lives."

—**Dr. Tana Dineen, author of *Manufacturing Victims***

"I think the book is terrific. I liked it because it supported a lot of the opinions I've had on psychiatry, cults, brainwashing and other ideas mentioned in the book."

—**Mort Walker**
Creator of *Beetle Bailey*
Founder and Chairman of
The International Museum of Cartoon Art

"Dozens of books have been written on the false memory problem that arises after vulnerable patients undergo suggestive therapy. But none is quite as charming as *Smiling Through Tears*. By skillfully interweaving professional cartoons with valuable information about the repressed memory controversy, therapy gone crazy and the power of suggestion, Freyd and Goldstein educate readers about one of the major problems in contemporary society. It's a must read not only for families that have been affected, but also for therapists and their patients; for educators and their students; and for people who care about people."

—**Elizabeth Loftus, Ph.D.**
Professor of Psychology, University of Washington
author of *The Myth of Repressed Memory*

A landmark case regarding repressed memories was reported on the front page of the New York Times on November 6, 1997.

Woman Wins Suit Claiming Therapists Invoked Traumatic Memories

By PAM BELLUCK

CHICAGO — While undergoing psychiatric therapy at a large Chicago hospital between 1986 and 1992, Patricia Burgus says, she was convinced by doctors that she had memories of being part of a satanic cult, of being sexually abused by numerous men, and of abusing her own two sons.

She says that hypnosis and other treatments caused her to believe she remembered cannibalizing people, so much so that her husband brought in a hamburger from a family picnic and therapists agreed to test the meat to see if it was human. Mrs. Burgus' sons were also hospitalized starting at the ages of 4 and 5, and subjected, she says, to disturbing therapy sessions, including one that involved seeing if they knew how to use handcuffs and a gun in an effort to verify what doctors suspected might be abusive incidents.

On Tuesday, lawyers for Mrs. Burgus said that insurance companies for two doctors and the hospital, Rush-Presbyterian-St. Luke's, had agreed to pay $10.6 million, the biggest settlement in a lawsuit alleging that therapists had invoked false memories and part of a growing legal backlash against therapies that try to elicit suppressed recollections.

Treatment that focuses on recovered memories gained popularity in the 1980s and over the last decade or so, recollections of abuse and other traumatic experiences have been the basis for civil lawsuits and even criminal cases. Six years ago, for example, a jury in Redwood City, Calif., convicted a man of raping and murdering a childhood playmate of his daughter in 1969, based largely on the latent recollections of the man's daughter.

But recently, the tide has been turning away from accepting the validity of these recovered memories.

Three years ago, the American Psychiatric Association cautioned that such memories were often not true and expressed skepticism about using hypnosis and other suggestive techniques to help elicit them. Judges have recently ruled to suppress court testimony from people who say they remembered abusive or criminal events under therapy. And a growing number of patients across the country have won lawsuits that accused therapists of leading them to recount false memories. At least 20 such suits have been filed in the last two years, with the plaintiffs successful in virtually all the ones that have been completed.

Last week, in Houston, a federal grand jury brought what are believed to be the first criminal charges in a case involving accusations that therapists induced false memories. The indictment charges that a hospital administrator and four therapists collected millions of dollars in fraudulent insurance payments by exaggerating patients' diagnoses and convincing them that they had been part of a satanic cult.

"This has been a craze that built up in the 1980s," said Dr. Paul R. McHugh, chairman of the department of psychiatry at the Johns Hopkins School of Medicine and an outspoken critic of the treatment, who was a consultant on Mrs. Burgus' case. "As in most cases, it has produced its damage and most people are coming to see the kinds of problems it represents. Could there have been someone who is abused and not remember it? I'm not saying that that's not possible. I'm saying first that these memories can never be validated without corroborating evidence. And secondly, it's a slippery slope opening the door for these conspiracy theories about satanic cults and alien abductions."

A spokesman for Rush-Presbyterian-St. Luke's Hospital, John Pontarelli, said officials there would not comment on the settlement, in which none of the parties admitted liability.

The psychiatrist who treated Mrs. Burgus' sons from 1986 to 1989, Dr. Elva Poznanski, the hospital's section chief of child and adolescent psychiatry, issued a statement saying, "On the basis of the knowledge available at that time, I would not change the treatment of these boys."

The other psychiatrist, Dr. Bennett G. Braun, director of the hospital's section of psychiatric trauma, said in an interview Tuesday that the settlement was a "travesty" and that his insurance company had settled the lawsuit despite his protestations that he had done nothing wrong.

Braun said: "A patient comes into the hospital doing so bad that she belongs in the hospital, and after several serious events in the hospital, which I can't disclose because of patient confidentiality, she was discharged and is doing much better. Where's the damage?"

Braun said that his treatment did not convince Mrs. Burgus of false memories. "She just spit it out," he said. "All of the cult stuff that she was talking about I learned from her. The idea to bring the meat in was hers. I merely said if he does bring it in, I will try to get it analyzed for human protein. Yes, the kids did see handcuffs. They did see a gun. But it was for therapeutic reasons."

He said Mrs. Burgus had exaggerated the use of hypnotism in treating her. "I'm not disagreeing with some of the things she says," Braun said. "It's just the slant."

Braun, 57, was the founding president of an organization called the International Society for the Study of Dissociation, which looks at theories of multiple personality and the idea that parts of the mind can dissociate certain experiences from other parts of the mind.

Dr. Elizabeth S. Bowman, an associate professor of psychiatry at the University of Indiana in Indianapolis and a past-president of the society, said that such therapists "firmly believe that people forget trauma, there's no question that memories return, and that some of the memories that return are accurate."

But she said that "the field has become more cautious because of lawsuits and we also with time are gaining more awareness that these memories sometimes are accurate and sometimes are not. We do try to educate patients about that."

Mrs. Burgus, 41, said in an interview that she became a patient at Rush-Presbyterian-St. Lukes in 1986, referred there by therapists in her hometown of Des Moines who had been treating her for what she describes as a severe post-partum depression following the difficult birth of her second son. She said she was diagnosed with multiple personality disorder and treated with various medications, hypnosis and, occasionally, kept in leather restraints, during six years of treatment, two and a half years as an inpatient. Her children were hospitalized, she said, because doctors believed her multiple personality disorder might be genetic.

She said she decided to file suit when, after getting out of the hospital, "I started to check out certain things that we had now based our lives on, these horror stories. I couldn't find any proof of anything."

Across the country in the last two years, other cases have been filed, many of them alleging similarly bizarre or violent memories. In 1995, a jury in Minnesota awarded $2.6 million to a woman who claimed her St. Paul psychiatrist told her that if she recovered her buried memories she would discover she had been sexually abused by relatives.

In 1996, a church in Springfield, Missouri agreed to pay $1 million to a woman who said that under the guidance of a church counselor, she came to believe that her father had raped her, got her pregnant and performed an abortion with a coat hanger—when in fact, she was still a virgin and her father had had a vasectomy. And in August, a jury awarded $5.8 million to a woman who claimed her psychotherapist implanted false memories of murder, satanic rituals, and cannibalism.

"The next thing I think there will be is legislation to force informed consent by psychiatric patients for this treatment," said Dr. R. Christopher Barden, a psychologist and a lawyer, who worked on Mrs. Burgus' case and said he has represented patients in about 20 such lawsuits. "I think insurance companies will stop reimbursing people for mental health treatments not proven safe and effective. This is the death knell for recovered memory therapy."

Smiling Through Tears
Table of Contents

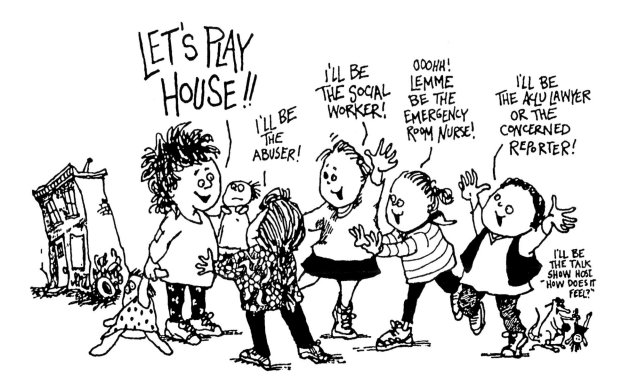

© 1996 Signe Wilkinson/Cartoonists & Writers Syndicate.

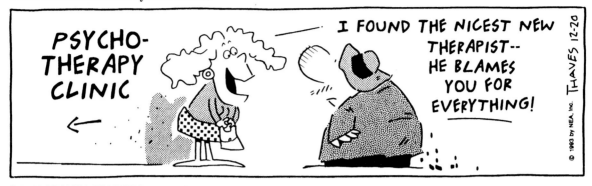

PSYCHO-
THERAPY
CLINIC
←

I FOUND THE NICEST NEW THERAPIST-- HE BLAMES YOU FOR EVERYTHING!

THAVES 12-20

© 1993 by NEA. INC.

An elderly couple lived through the Holocaust in Poland where they met as children in a concentration camp. They say, "this is worse."

A father of three glanced out of the window as his young daughter ran across the street. She was killed by a speeding car. He says the anguish now is worse.

A grandmother whose entire family had to leave Austria in the 1940s, penniless and fearful of losing their lives under fascism, says she is more tortured now.

A mother suffered several years with a daughter dying of leukemia. She says her life is more miserable now than it was then.

What is causing this indescribable misery for parents whose past experiences seem less significant than the tragedies they are now suffering? Their adult children have accused them of horrendous crimes that the parents say never happened.

What would you do if you were accused of a crime that you did not commit? How would you respond if the child who you nurtured and nourished suddenly accused you of abuse that you did not commit and then refused to speak to you, severing contact with anyone who did not agree with the accusations?

Stunned? Humiliated? Angry?

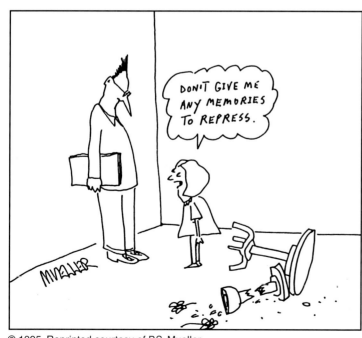

DON'T GIVE ME ANY MEMORIES TO REPRESS.

MUELLER

Wouldn't you have these feelings? Wouldn't you want to understand what was happening? Wouldn't you want to try to defend yourself against such treatment?

Searching for answers, families have consulted experts, immersed themselves in memory research, and joined support organizations. What these families have discovered is that they and their children are victims of junk therapy.

At the end of the 1980s, something unparalleled gripped our nation. The "survivor" movement was born. An outgrowth of the "recovery" movement, it was propelled by such books as *The Courage to Heal* (1988), *Toxic Parents* (1989) and *Secret Survivors* (1990). Gender feminists, New Age proponents and recovery enthusiasts also promoted this movement.

Typically, the accusers were middle-class, adult women between the ages of 25 and 50; but many teens and men also consider themselves survivors. These survivors

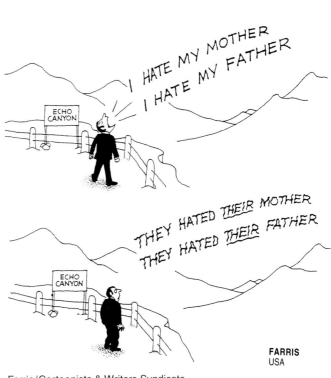

Farris/Cartoonists & Writers Syndicate

claimed that they had "recovered repressed memories" of sadistic and perverse acts of sexual abuse and physical cruelty, memories they had "repressed" since childhood.

Claiming amnesia, survivors maintained that they "dissociated" and thus were protected from the "torture that was their

NON SEQUITUR

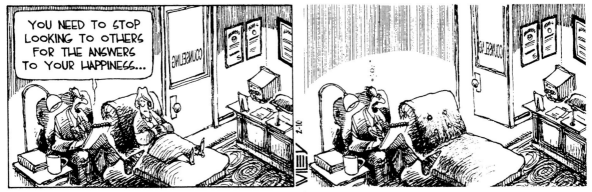

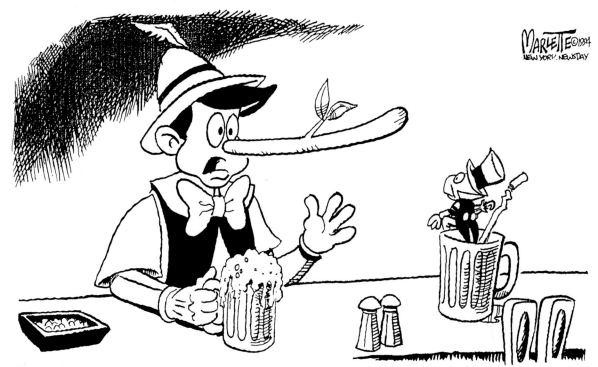

"I WASN'T EXACTLY *LYING!*... I THOUGHT IT WAS A *REPRESSED MEMORY!*... BUT POOR OLD *GEPPETTO* GOT SENT UP ON A *MORALS CHARGE!*"

childhood" until they discovered a "safe place" in therapy, where the memories were "retrieved."

Authors of recovery books suggest that "if you think you were abused and your life shows the symptoms, then you were."[1] Parents who denied such bizarre accusations were told that their denial was proof of their guilt. Lacking corroborating evidence, survivors alleged that the indisputable proof of their abuse was the fact that they had forgotten—until "therapy."

Since the early 1990s, dozens of books and hundreds of articles have been written describing this cruel attack on families, now more commonly referred to as False Memory Syndrome (FMS). By 1993, cartoons about repressed memories and False Memory Syndrome began to appear, an indication that the general public was becoming aware of these issues. Through humor, cartoonists have captured the social implications of this phenomenon. Before a cartoon can be appreciated, a reader must be aware and understand a critical amount of information—otherwise the cartoon will not elicit a response.

During the past several years, we have amassed hundreds of cartoons on False Memory Syndrome and the trends that have converged to nurture its growth. We think the cartoons tell an interesting story about an issue unprecedented in history. Because the major social movements that evolved during the 1980s and early 1990s are now more widely recognized, cartoonists are able to communicate and bring meaning to this crisis.

In the ordinary course of life, people come to accept that tragedies occur: loved ones become sick and sometimes die; debilitating accidents happen; and sometimes children suffer terrible fates. We know that war and famines and hurricanes and floods occur, and that we are helpless in the face of those disasters. We strive to understand and cope with an imperfect world.

As we become educated we try to control our destiny. We teach our children the difference between right and wrong, hoping our children will be "good and happy people" above all else. In our culture, we also say that the worst thing a parent can experience is the death of a child. Now, tens of thousands of parents say there is something almost as devastating. Some have said it is even worse because of a lack of closure. They have lost a child, but there is no mourning, no ritual for grieving, no sympathy from friends.

MORE FUN WITH POST-THERAPY DISORDER

Instead, they live in dread, fearful of what their misguided children might say or do that will harm themselves and their families.

We have listened to thousands of these parents from every state in the United States and other English-speaking nations. We have met with parents who are dazed at having lost the love and respect of their children; parents who have been degraded, humiliated, embarrassed or even imprisoned; parents whose lives have been shattered by their own children! All the good things between these parents and their children destroyed—their lives have been trashed.

We have helped to describe and document a phenomenon that has become epidemic in the decade of the nineties: False Memory Syndrome. We have wrestled with this issue for more than five years and have begun to understand why adult children, who once loved their parents, have abandoned them in a desperate effort to hold on to a false belief.

We are fully aware of the extent of child abuse and of the terrible consequences that abuse may cause. Society should not tolerate such abhorrent behavior.

False accusations of abuse, however, exacerbate the problem of child abuse by creating doubt about all claims and drain-

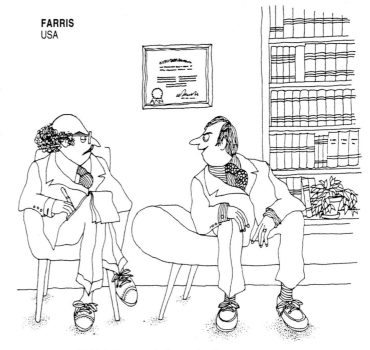

FARRIS
USA

"I think I'm cured. I now forgive my parents, love my wife, adore my children and hate you."

Farris/Cartoonists & Writers Syndicate

ing scarce financial, legal and emotional resources from children who need them now.

This book is about the misuse of dangerous mind-altering techniques and about the social trends that have nurtured their use in therapy.

Child abuse is a problem. False accusations brought only on the basis of claims of recovered repressed memories are a problem. They are separate problems and both need to be solved in the cause of justice.

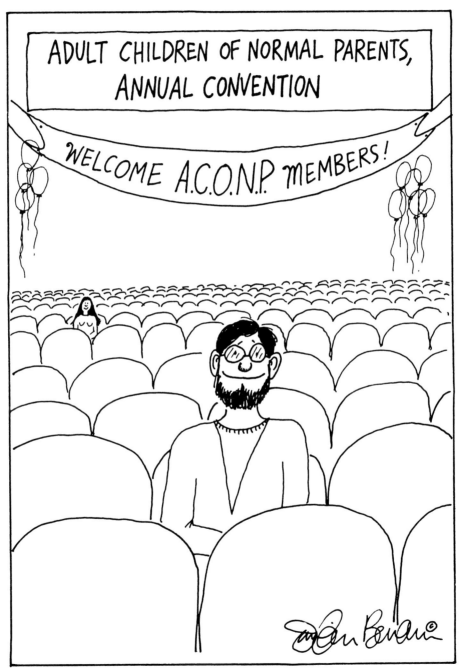

Reprinted with permission from Jennifer Berman.

Your family is dysfunctional! According to recovery guru, John Bradshaw and other pop psychologists, nearly 100% of families in the United States are dysfunctional. Don't laugh, being labeled dysfunctional is serious business.

It means that the family needs therapy. In fact, every family member needs therapy because the abuse that exists in dysfunctional families is codependent and intergenerational. According to the dogma, it will take five generations to heal the abuse,[1] and healing can only take place under the guidance of a therapist.

If a person doesn't recognize that his or her family is dysfunctional, that is an example of being "in denial." Often the father is labeled the "perpetrator" and the mother the "enabler." These roles may be reversed. Parents are accused of committing heinous crimes—the physical, emotional and sexual abuse of *their own child*.

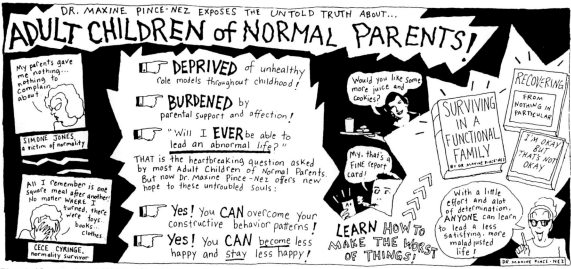

Piccolo/Cartoonists & Writers Syndicate

PICCOLO Toronto CANADA

Calvin and Hobbes

by Bill Watterson

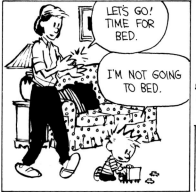
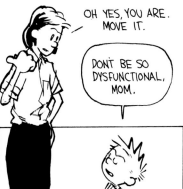
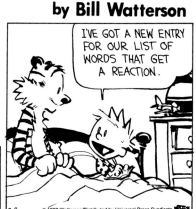

What is a dysfunctional family anyway?

In the last few decades, the family has been redefined. Much interpretation of family dynamics takes place in self-help groups and in therapists' offices. In such settings, parents are often judged and condemned by people who don't even know them. In a self-help group or therapist's office only one side of a family scenario is presented, often by a person who is distraught, depressed and desperately seeking answers to life's problems. As Carl Sagan has noted, the role of the therapist in this type of therapy is to validate the patient.

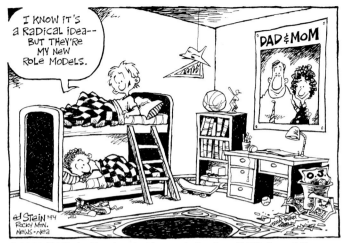

© 1994 Ed Stein. Reprinted with permission from Ed Stein and Newspaper Enterprise Association.

The thing I've been most appalled by is the sense of so many psychotherapists . . . that their job is to confirm their patients' delusions rather than help them find out what really has happened. It took a long time to convince myself that's what's happening, but it certainly is happening. I don't know whether it's more likely among social workers than Ph.D.s in psychology, or more likely among the Ph.D.s than the psychiatrists, who have medical training. But I do find it astonishing that anybody in psychology should be ignorant of the most elementary precepts of skeptical scientific scrutiny.

As someone who spent a lot of time reading Freud and his followers, I also am distressed by the absence of a systematic effort to demonstrate that psychoanalysis is more useful than going to your priest or rabbi. Or whether there is such a thing as repression. It's always very dangerous when the error-correcting machinery is not working and there aren't systematic attempts to disprove what the revered founder of your field maintains.[2]

The current generation of adult children came of age during a tumultuous time in history when some unusual ideas were afloat. These ideas made them vulnerable to dangerous trends. Trends that later became significant movements.

In the 1980s and 1990s, tens of thousands of families who believed they were normal now discovered they were dysfunctional. The concept of the wounded adult child emerged. Myriads of adults were taught to think of themselves as adult children with a wounded inner child. The "adult child" was then led on a journey to explore his or her past and hunt for abusers.

The belief that most families are dysfunctional was so prevalent that hundreds of books were written on the subject and thousands of self-help groups formed to overcome the effects of the dysfunctional family. The underlying assumption is that every problem an adult child faces in life—whether it be an eating disorder, depression, trouble with relationships, difficulty with jobs—is the result of poor parenting. Responsibility shifts from the adult child and blame is placed on mom and dad.

The survivor dogma holds that the terrible torture experienced during childhood leads the victim to dissociate and repress memories, sometimes for several decades. In order for healing to occur, the memories must be recalled, often through the use of hypnosis or other mind-altering techniques.

When the memory is recalled, so goes the theory, the perpetrator must be identified and perhaps confronted. Typically, relationships and contacts are immediately severed with anyone who does not believe the accuser's story.

Memories conjured up during misdirected therapy become the foundation for false accusations—devastating families, destroying reputations and depleting finances. The mental anguish of those falsely accused and relentlessly persecuted is indescribable.

The families that we met appear to be successful members of society. They are well-educated, upper middle-class, morally forthright, caring people. Yet, they have been targeted as dysfunctional. Surveys taken of these families indicate that for the most part they followed the practices of what is considered good parenting. Generally, they had dinner together as a family; went on trips together (parents and children); attended church as a family; engaged in extended family activities, such as reunions with grandparents, uncles and aunts; and attended school activities. However, according to the dysfunctional family theory, parents in such families are often controlling, manipulative and demanding with high expectations that demean the child.

Today, within the recovery-oriented culture, the dysfunctional label is applied to most families, and as some critics have pointed out, "Blaming parents for what they did or didn't do has become a national obsession—and big business."[3]

THE BUCKETS

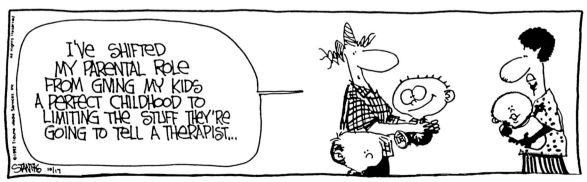

FEIFFER®

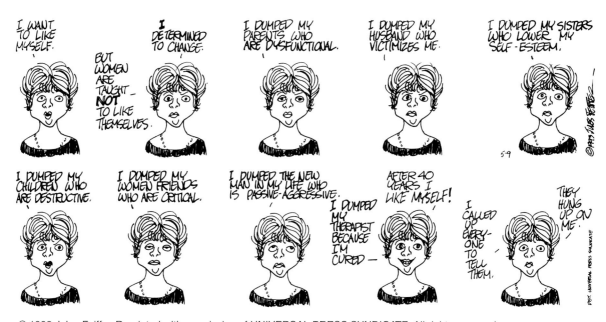

Several times I* have been on a platform with Gloria Steinem at meetings of the American Library Association. She was the main speaker, and I was either the presenter or recipient of an award for activities in the area of intellectual freedom.

Gloria has been introduced as one of the ten most influential women in America. Yet, she has claimed that she lacked self-esteem. She claims that if she had more self-esteem, she perhaps would have been a lawyer. She would have reached even greater pinnacles of success.

Her book, *Revolution From Within: A Book of Self-Esteem*, argues that low self-esteem is responsible for almost every evil on earth. According to Gloria and many other feminists, our society is a patriarchy and little girls learn low self-esteem at an early age from their parents, teachers and religious leaders. Gloria says:

The little girl who is discouraged from strength and exploring, or is punished for willfullness and praised for assuming a docility and smiling sweetness she doesn't feel, often begins to construct a "deflated" self, which results in the mostly female problem of depression.[1]

Correlating with the feminist movement, the self-esteem movement began in the 1960s. The feminists dealt with many goals that most of us, who consider ourselves to be fair-minded men or women, heartily agree. Some aspects of the movement, however, became shockingly combative, especially the claim that all men are basically rapists and intentionally raped their daughters so they would maintain their subservient roles as the docile and obedient future wives of America.

When feminists looked to the history of their subjugation they came to believe that women's problems were the fault of men, since men have always been in control. And what did men do to keep women under control? Why they raped, humiliated and shamed them. Therefore, women have low self-esteem. According to the rhetoric, even

Eleanor Goldstein is the author of this chapter.

Calvin and Hobbes

by Bill Watterson

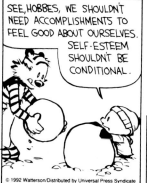

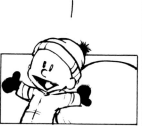

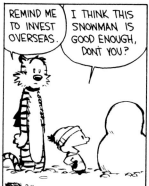

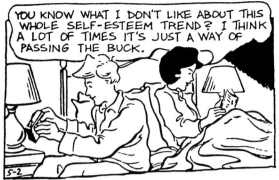 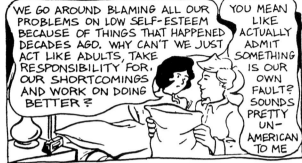

successful women have low self esteem. The reason these women are successful is to overcome their low self-esteem.

Supporting the theory that childhood abuse contributes to low self-esteem are such celebrities as Marilyn Van Derbur and Roseanne Barr.

Van Derbur says that she was abused from age 5 to age 18 years but she was unaware of it until she was 24 years old. She states that she became a "day child" who was an over-achiever and a "night child" who was sexually abused.

The abuse caused Van Derbur to suffer from low self-esteem. She compensated by becoming perfect in every way. She was a four-point student at the University of Colorado, where one of her professors told me that Marilyn was the smartest student he ever had. I was in the same class, entitled "Man in the Physical World." I reminded Marilyn about that class about a year ago when we spoke on the phone. She had forgotten me, the class and the professor. However, her restored memories are very vivid.

I went to visit Roseanne's parents in Salt Lake City. Roseanne claims that she had low self-esteem because she was overweight and misunderstood, growing up Jewish in a community of Mormons. Her parents were and still are loved and accepted in that community. Roseanne claims to have been abused while her mother changed her diaper. She remembers her father peeking into the bathroom while she bathed. Her father showed me the bathroom; there is no place to peek through.

What achievements would these women have made, if only they had not been so irretrievably damaged as children and thus forced to grow up with low self-esteem? According to Steinem:

> When core self-esteem remains low even into adulthood, no amount of external task-oriented achievement or approval seems able to compensate . . . which is why a lack of core self-esteem can produce totalitarian leaders for whom no amount of power is enough . . . and authoritarian parents for whom no obedience is complete.[2]

Dozens of characteristics have been blamed on poor self-esteem including being angry, impatient, hotheaded, sarcastic, jealous, violent, hateful, cruel, unfriendly, vain, insensitive, unethical, lazy, rude, unforgiving and depressed. According to the self-esteem movement, if you have any of the above characteristics, you probably have low self-esteem. And your low self-esteem stems from being abused as a child, probably by your father, mother, or other trusted family member, or maybe a teacher or neighbor.

Self-esteem became a political movement in the 1990s and many state legislatures mandated that teachers take courses about self-esteem and incorporate lessons in the classroom. In support of the self-esteem movement, California State Assemblyman John Vasconcellos commented: "What splitting the atom had been to the 1940s and exploring outer space had been to the 1960s, exploring 'the reaches and mysteries of inner space' would become to the 1990s."[3]

There was a significant response by parents and teachers to the self-esteem movement. Many became afraid to correct or discipline children for fear they would harm the child's self-esteem. The idea of accepting a person for who he or she was, meant that criticism was out of place. Only positive reinforcement was considered acceptable.

Was the result an overdose of self-esteem that is not warranted or deserved? Many children grew up thinking they knew more than anyone else, including their parents. These children had little respect for their parents. They expected that since they were so smart, life would be great in every respect. Many were headed for disappointment as they did not live up to their own expectations. When these feelings led to therapy, they learned that they were blameless for the mishaps in their lives, they learned that their problems were due to low self-esteem created by an abusive family and living in a patriarchal society.

Rather than encouraging one to take responsibility, recovered memory therapy encourages one to look to the past and consider oneself as a victim.

Self-esteem overdose dangerous, experts say

By LEAH GARCHIK
San Francisco Chronicle

It's possible that you think too much of yourself.

Common wisdom has had it that a lack of self-esteem is the biggest problem facing young people, criminals, the depressed, the abused, the abusers and everyone else who doesn't go around with a smiley face pinned to his lapel. Now comes *Health* magazine, which reports on studies showing that there is such a thing as too much self-esteem.

At the University of California at UC Riverside, students who gave themselves ratings above those of their observers on cheerfulness, warmth and intelligence were perceived to be hostile, deceitful and condescending. The conclusions of psychologist David Funder eerily echo the kitchen wisdom of mothers long before psychologists were conducting such tests: When you raise yourself higher than the view others have of you, "you think you're wonderful and other people think you're a creep."

Psychologist Roy Baumeister at Case Western Reserve University contradicts the common wisdom by insisting that crimes more often are a result of inflated rather than deflated self-esteem.

Baumeister decries a "general inflation of self-worth in our culture. It's time for society as a whole to be a little more humble."[4]

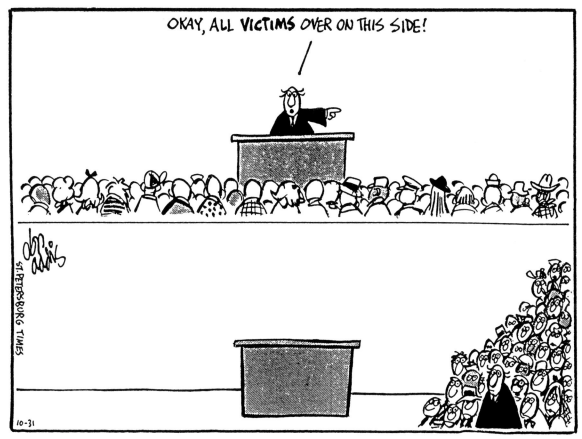

Ours is a culture that at one time idolized the strength, courage and independence of cowboys. Hollywood glamorized heroes such as Buffalo Bill and Wyatt Earp of the Old West. Movies were made and silver screen role models John Wayne, Roy Rogers and Clint Eastwood were created. These public figures inspired a generation, but times have changed. Today's society has shifted to a culture of victims where recovery champions proudly boast, "I am a survivor."

The civil rights movement and the feminist movement brought needed public attention to the injustices suffered by many. Victims' rights became a rallying point for women and African Americans seeking equality and justice. Native Americans, the physically handicapped and many other minority groups created their own movements. The fact that children were often abused became acknowledged and advocates organized to protect children.

If children are commonly abused today, it became the dogma both that many adult

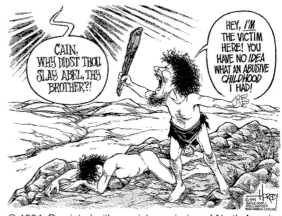

children must have been abused in the past and that their lives showed the symptoms—even if the memories of abuse were forgotten. These ideas spread as books were written claiming that children commonly forget the abuse they suffer. In addition, the statutes of limitations in sexual abuse cases were amended allowing victims of childhood sexual abuse to bring lawsuits against their perpetrators. This opened the door for people to file lawsuits based on "recovered and repressed memories."

As public concern and discourse for

Calvin and Hobbes   by Bill Watterson

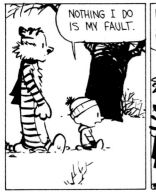

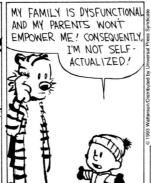

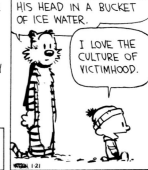

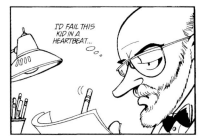
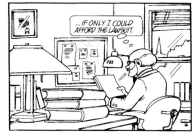
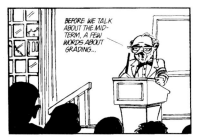
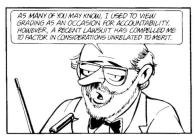
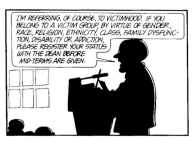
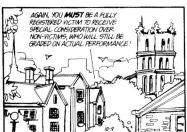
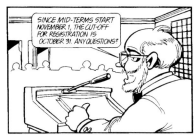
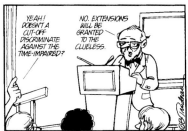

victims grew, more funding became available and an increasing number of groups began to define themselves as victims. Victimology not only entered our vernacular, it penetrated our societal beliefs and norms. Dr. Tana Dineen, in her new book, *Manufacturing Victims*, comments on this phenomenon:

> *"Victim," once a term reserved for those who suffered from a calamity of nature, of Fate or of violent crime, now has become psychologized so that it can be applied broadly to anyone and everyone. . . . Symptoms such as unhappiness, boredom, anger, sadness, and guilt, can now all be interpreted as signs of prior trauma, creating victims. Whether these people then pursue treatment, sue their perpetrator, or seek other victims for support, they all become "users" of the Psychology Industry, providing its income and increasing its overall asset worth.*[1]

In the early 1990s, celebrities began speaking about abusive childhoods, exposing to the public that they came from abusive families. These celebrities seemed to have reached the American dream—fame, fortune, living the lifestyle of the rich and famous as their careers soared. Marilyn Van Derbur, Roseanne, Latoya Jackson and many others define themselves and their life's work as "survivors" of childhood abuse.

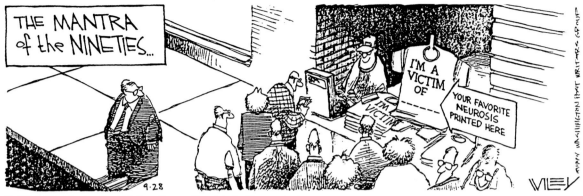

As victims, people found explanations to the normal disappointments, tragedies and hardships of life. Not only could being a victim be profitable in terms of suing your parents and their hefty homeowner policy, but it also became fashionable. The recovery movement has accomplished what no other movement has been able to achieve: it extended the definition of victimhood to encompass fabricated victims and it bestowed glamour on survivorship. As one critic pointed out: "In the 1990s, everyone wants to be a survivor, as if survivalhood were the only alternative to victimization."[2]

Victimhood has become a celebrated identity in our society. Within the recovery-oriented culture, almost everyone claimed to be a victim of familial abuse. Dysfunctional families are the culprits, recovery experts claim, and "victimology can fairly be called the study of our culture."[3] If life is unfair, you are a victim. If you've had a string of bad relationships, you are a victim. If your parent(s) were overprotective, if you cannot lose weight, if you are dissatisfied at work or at home, you are a victim.

Why then, would people allow themselves to be categorized as "victims?" Why would anyone knowingly want this label? Evidently, being a victim seems to be a coveted identity in today's society. The appeal to this is a quick fix and no responsibility: an identity that is much revered, despite the fact that being labeled as such reduces women to children and society as a whole to hapless, helpless victims.

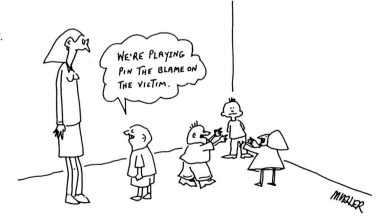

My recovery is going GREAT!

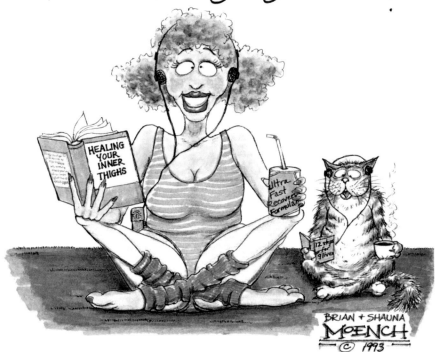

I'm working my program, attending my meetings and doing the 12 steps. I'm in touch with my feelings, reclaiming my personal power and healing my inner child. I meditate, play my "self talk" tapes and I'm becoming one with the universe.... Now if I could just remember what it is I'm recovering from.......

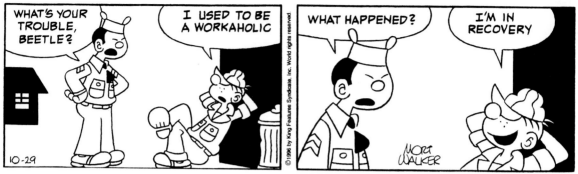

Is an alcoholic a sinner, criminal or victim? Is an alcoholic suffering from a disease, a weak personality or past abuse? Millions of people are alcoholics and the way alcoholism is defined determines the treatment they will receive.

Will he or she be sent to a church, hospital, prison, rehab center, Alcoholics Anonymous (AA) group or therapy? Wherever the alcoholic seeks help or is sent for treatment, he or she will most likely be part of a 12-Step program.

The 12 Steps are the cornerstone of virtually every self-help recovery program in the United States. Furthermore, almost every institution that purports to help addicts overcome their addictions is based on the 12-Step model.

What are the 12 Steps? How did they originate? What influence do they have on modern culture?

The 12 Steps originated under the umbrella of the Oxford Group Movement that was founded by Dr. Frank Nathan Daniel Buchman, who was born in 1878. In 1902, Buchman graduated from Mount Airy Seminary in Pennsylvania and was ordained

as a Lutheran Minister. His belief system, which permeated his teachings, was to rely on the guidance of God in all aspects of life. During the early period of the Oxford Group Movement certain ideas emerged.[1]

These basic ideas were:

1) *both public and private confession of sin, with an emphasis upon sexual sin;*

2) *reception of divine "guidance" during "quiet times";*

3) *complete surrender to this "guidance";*

4) *the living of a "guided" life in which every aspect of one's actions, down to the choice of dinner entree, was controlled by God;*

5) *practice of the Buchmanite "four absolutes"–purity, honesty, love, and unselfishness.*[2]

The founders of AA, Bill Wilson and Dr. Robert Smith (Dr. Bob), were both alcoholics whose drinking so affected their lives that they could not function normally. After decades of drinking and numerous crises, Bill was admitted to Town's Hospital in 1934. There he had a spiritual awakening while under the influence of a hallucinogen (belladonna), which was used as a treatment at the hospital.

He described the experience in Alcoholics Anonymous Comes of Age:

I found myself crying out, "If there is a God, let Him show Himself! I am ready to do anything!"

Suddenly the room lit up with a great white light. . . . All about me there was a wonderful feeling of Presence, and I thought to myself, "So this is the God of the Preachers."[3]

In 1935, Dr. Bob, a skilled surgeon, a hardcore alcoholic and an adherent of the Oxford Group Movement was introduced to Bill Wilson. Bill and Bob had intended to meet for just a few minutes but spent more than six hours talking. Soon Bob moved into Bill's home where the practice of the Oxford Group principles became the focus of their lives. From then on, Bob and Bill spent most of their efforts "working on" other drunks. June 10, 1935, is often cited as the founding date of Alcoholics Anonymous.[4]

In the Spring of 1938, Bill Wilson began writing the *Big Book* of AA. The 12 Steps as described in the book were a distillation of the Oxford Group Movement principles. Almost every single one of the 12 Steps can be traced back to the Oxford Group principles.[5]

In May 1938, the newly formed organization of AA was set up to unite the group and enable the wealthy to give tax-deductible donations. The *Big Book* was published in April 1939, with a press run of 5,000 copies. AA had about 100 members at that time.[6]

On March 1, 1941, the *Saturday Evening Post* published an article about AA, which brought considerable recognition to the organization. As a result of the article about 6,000 people joined AA.[7]

In the final days of 1941, A.A. had 200 groups, a membership of 8,000, and a national office in New York City. By 1944, A.A. had 360 groups with a total membership of 10,000, and in June of that year had begun publication of what was to become its official organ, The Grapevine, *which had originally been a newsletter for A.A.s in the armed forces.*[8]

Today, AA is a mass organization. Worldwide, there are over 80,000 groups.[9] Over

Nancy

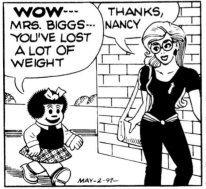
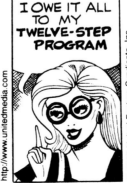
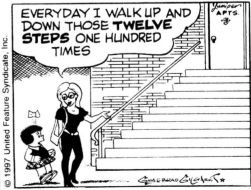

BENT OFFERINGS   by Don Addis

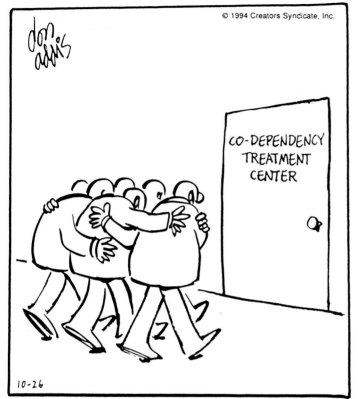

© 1994 Creators Syndicate, Inc.

CO-DEPENDENCY
TREATMENT
CENTER

10-26

© 1994 Don Addis. Reprinted with permission from Don Addis and Creators Syndicate, Inc.

tory of *themselves* and admit *their* "wrongs?"

The message and the format of 12-Step programs is so appealing to so many people that it has spawned the proliferation of dozens of imitative groups. There now are 12-Step programs for everyone—overeaters, gamblers, sex addicts, in addition to children, friends and spouses of addicts—for example.

In addition to AA, codependency became part of the recovery movement.

Codependence, which originally referred to the problems of women married to alcoholics, was discovered by pop psychologists and addiction counselors during the 1980s and redefined. Now it applies to any problem associated with an addiction, real or imagined, suffered by you or someone close to you. Now this amorphous disease is a business.[10]

the years, the 12-Step program has not changed at all. What is surprising is the large number of groups that have adopted the 12 Steps, even when apparently inappropriate. The most extreme example is Incest Survivors Anonymous.

If the AA program (the 12 Steps) was truly tailored to suit the needs of alcoholics (or addicts of any sort), it would seem grotesque that it be adopted as the program for "victims" of hideous and cruel crimes. Should victims really adopt guiding principles as stated in the 12 Steps that emphasize that *they* should make "amends" to those *they've* "harmed," take a moral inven-

The sinner and disease model of treatment has largely succumbed to the recovery model. In this model, the therapist may be the higher power and the victim becomes a survivor. In the recovery movement, the victim is absolved from personal responsibility, thus shifting from the sinner to the survivor. The survivor is a victim. What is he or she a victim of? Abuse—probably at the hands of Mom or Dad. Thus, the search for perpetrators began.

22

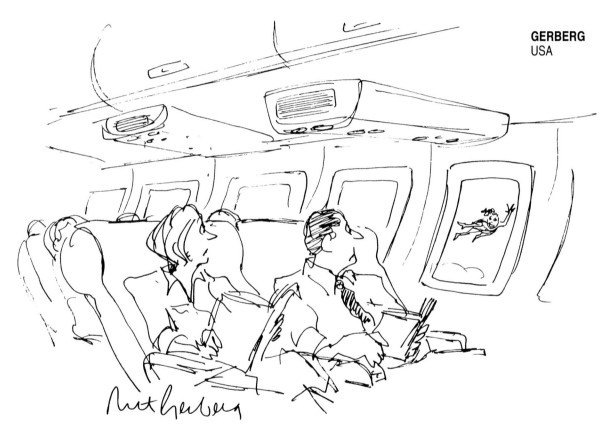

GERBERG
USA

" . . . This is the captain again. We're now at 30,000 feet cruising over the Rockies,
and if you look out the left side of the aircraft you may catch a glimpse
of Shirley MaClaine, who's having a brief out-of-body experience."

Gerberg/Cartoonists & Writers Syndicate

New Age provides a huge umbrella for a potpourri of ideas. Visit your local bookstore. Under New Age you will find books on the following topics: astrology, psychics, acupuncture, crystals, moon signs, dream interpretation, Oriental mythology, magic, ghosts, gemstones, goddesses, sun signs, astrocycles, out-of-body experience, Tao of symbols, creative visualization, Tarot cards, astral projection, hypnotism, fortune telling, UFOs, paranormal experience, auras, ESP, healing, focusing, life-extension, age regression, reincarnation, channeling, homeopathy, mind-body connection, macrobiotics and more. The authors range from the uncredentialed to Ph.D.s from some of our most prestigious universities. It does not seem to matter.

What ties New Age thinking together so that these diverse ideas fit under one umbrella? Maybe it is the fact that the ideas do not fit anywhere else. The topics in these books could not be categorized under the more traditional, recognized disciplines such as science, health, psychology or philosophy. Therefore, if they do not fit anywhere else, it's New Age.

The common theme that New Age topics seem to share is a lack of trust in the scientific method to determine answers or results. Instead, they rely on feelings, intuition, imagination, hearsay and superstition—forget logic, data, analysis or the need for replication in an unbiased setting.

Some proponents of the New Age movement assume that rational, scientific investigation into the mysteries of the mind, body and universe is inadequate and outdated. New Age adherents subscribe to a "new consciousness," characterized by mystical beliefs in such things as magic, astrology, numerology, the occult, sorcery and shamans. Influenced partly by Eastern mysticism, New Age offers the promise of achieving "self-actualization" and reaching a higher "consciousness" through meditation, yoga and holistic body healing. Magical charms, ancient myths and the healing powers of crystals and pyramids are prevalent in this belief system. Out-of-body experiences, past-life regression and contact with spirits from other dimensions are readily accepted.

Many of the adult children who have

HAGAR THE HORRIBLE

CHRIS BROWNE

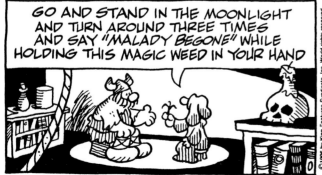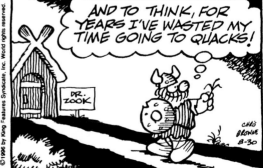

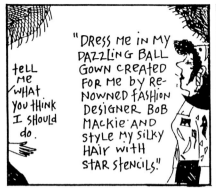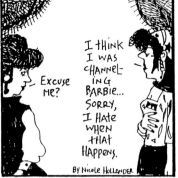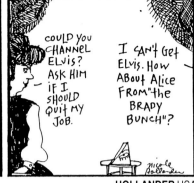

"DRESS ME IN MY DAZZLING BALL GOWN CREATED FOR ME by RENOWNED FASHION DESIGNER BOB MACKIE AND STYLE MY SILKY HAIR WITH STAR STENCILS."

tell me WHAT you think I SHOULD do.

Excuse me?

I THINK I WAS CHANNELING BARBIE... SORRY, I HATE WHEN THAT HAPPENS.

BY NICOLE HOLLANDER

COULD YOU CHANNEL ELVIS? ASK HIM IF I SHOULD QUIT MY JOB.

I CAN'T GET ELVIS. HOW ABOUT ALICE FROM "THE BRADY BUNCH"?

Hollander/Cartoonists & Writers Syndicate

HOLLANDER USA

recovered repressed memories of childhood abuse are proponents of New Age ideas.

How did New Age ideas influence these women? New Age supposedly provides answers to everything: nutrition, health, the great philosophical questions of who we are, where we were and where we are going. Gurus of New Age thinking claim to have "the" answers. Finding peace within oneself as a prelude to planetary harmony is one goal of New Age thinking. Neo-paganism, witchcraft, goddesses and Druids offer religious alternatives to the traditional Western religious beliefs.

New Age techniques include visualization, imaging, chanting, meditation, fasting, sensory deprivation, hypnosis and body massage. These techniques can all have a profound impact on thought processes. In addition to the many New Age seminars, groups and books, there are tapes as well. The tapes are hypnotic, many claiming to carry subliminal messages. And how significant can subliminal messages be? We just don't know.

New Age has become very influential in the United States. One president was known to be influenced by astrology, some movie stars have used channeling and other well-admired celebrities use these and countless other New Age techniques.

Why is New Age dangerous? It ignores science and believes intuition is as good as evidence. Though some aspects may be positive, the danger lies in relying only on a New Age approach in response to health and other problems.

What happens when an adherent, who depends on New Age thinking for the answers to life, has something go wrong?

GOULD
USA

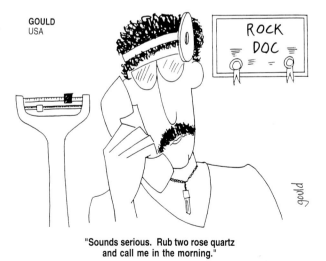

"Sounds serious. Rub two rose quartz and call me in the morning."

Gould/Cartoonists & Writers Syndicate

Who is to blame? Certainly not the person herself or himself, the guru or the New Age concept. The problem has to be outside of that person—something done to her or him. This is where New Age meets the survivor movement. For many, New Age techniques—such as age regression—become the prescribed therapy, providing the path for recovered memories. Through visualization, imaging or hypnosis, answers can be found. Generally, it is a parent or other caretaker, not the New Age proponent, who is considered at fault for the problem.

New Age healers reject modern medicine and view cancer, multiple sclerosis (MS) and diabetes as having psychological origins. Healing of such illnesses can only take place with therapy or imaging away the illness. With this mindset it is easy to see how parents come to be blamed for their adult children's problems. If therapy, hypnotism or visualizations do not discover the person (in this life) who is the culprit, then regress or channel to a previous life—because that's where the problem may lie.

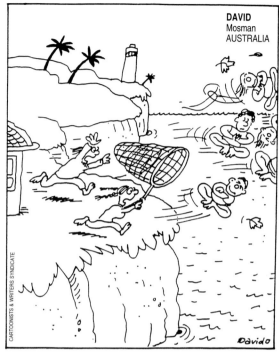

AT THE NIRVANA SCHOOL OF ENLIGHTENMENT AN UNFORTUNATE OFFSHORE BREEZE WIPES OUT HALF THE LEVITATION CLASS.

David/Cartoonists & Writers Syndicate

Since science and non-science are mixed in unequal proportions, the New Age movement provides a breeding ground in which confabulations can thrive.

NON SEQUITUR

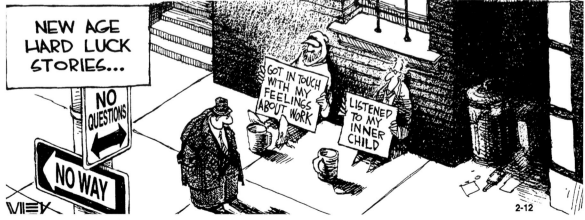

© 1997, Washington Post Writers Group. Reprinted with permission.

DENNIS THE MENACE

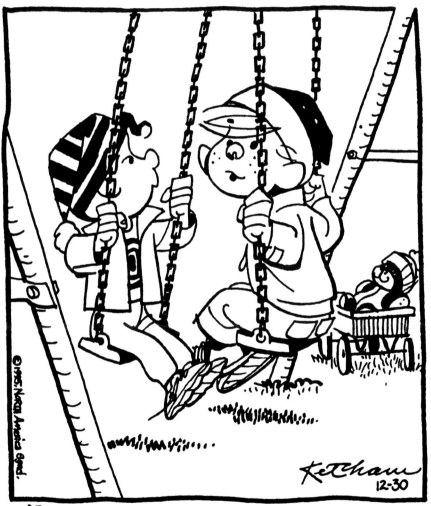

"IMAGINATION IS WHAT LETS YOU REMEMBER THINGS THAT *NEVER* HAPPENED, JOEY."

DENNIS THE MENACE® used by permission of Hank Ketcham and © 1995 by North America Syndicate.

The recovery movement is built on the mistaken belief that minds are like tape recorders and every experience is recorded someplace in the brain. Part of this belief system holds that traumatic memory is special. The presumption is that a trauma is so horrible it cannot be dealt with. It is transferred someplace else in the brain and becomes a repressed memory. Repressed memories are believed to fester and cause damage to a person until the memory is retrieved and confronted. There is not a shred of evidence for this theory.

Disagreements within the memory research community are not new. There have been strong arguments about whether there are single or multiple memory systems, for example.[1] But the kind of acrimony that has been part of the "memory wars" about validity of repressed memories has been unusual and surprising. There are, however, many basic ideas about memory on which there is agreement.

As long ago as 1932, Frederic Bartlett showed that memory is reconstructed and that it can be influenced by many things such as our attitudes, our current expectations and our concerns.[2] When we have a memory, we take bits and pieces and reconstruct a story that makes sense to us in the here and now, rather like filling in the blanks. Sometimes our memories are historically accurate, sometimes our memories are a mixture of accurate and inaccurate information and sometimes they are false. That is true whether the memory is continuous or whether it is remembered after a time of having been forgotten.

Most of us are uncomfortable with the thought that we could have false memories because, after all, we are our memories. We are who we are in terms of what we remember about ourselves. It goes against reason to think that we could be who we are if our

Doonesbury G.B. Trudeau

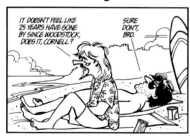
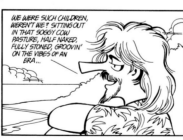
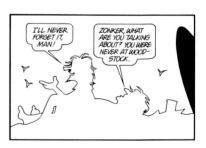
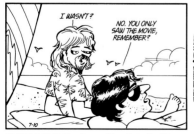
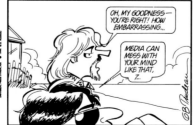
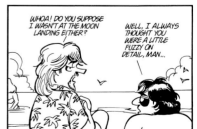

Shoe

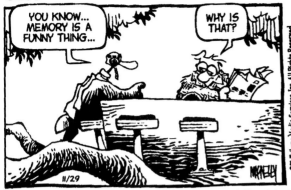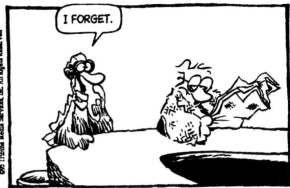

memories could be false. It seems impossible that *we* could have false memories, although we might think that *others* do. If we can't trust our own memories, then what can we trust?

Mostly, our memories do a good job for us. We are descendants of people who remembered where the dangers in the forest lurked. If they had not remembered, they would likely have been gobbled up.

In our daily lives we normally don't think about memory. Like language, it's just there. Before there was written language, people drew pictures on cave walls to help them remember the past. They incorporated stories into verse as an aid to recall. Even today, people take photographs and buy souvenirs as aids to remember special experiences. Some take notes and tape events to help them remember. Whatever we may think or say about our memories, we often act in ways that indicate our memory is fallible and our memories may fade.

While literature is filled with references to fading memories—whether mixed with desire or woven with dreams—in the past few decades, the notion of memory as a

videotape recorder or as a computer came to shape the metaphors that we use for it today. A belief emerged that our experiences are recorded like images on film or bits of information in the computer. This notion was bolstered by the research of Wilder Penfield whose electric probes into the brains of some epilepsy patients seemed to stimulate memories. The fantastic nature of some of these memories, however, was one clue that he had not shown memory operated like a device, recording everything.[3]

Memory research has demonstrated that only some of the information we perceive and experience is put into memory and sometimes what is saved is not entirely accurate. For example, have you ever had the experience of returning to a favorite childhood spot only to find that it is much smaller than you remembered—a child's perspective. Once information is stored in memory it is also subject to fading or even loss. New information sometimes interferes with our memory when we try to remember something. Elizabeth Loftus' research, which focuses on eyewitness testimony has shown that what people think they have seen can be influenced simply in the way a question is asked. Did you see *a* broken headlight? or Did you see *the* broken headlight? can change what some people think they remember.[4]

The development of new technologies allowing us to see the sections of the brain that are activated when people think, have helped to show that the brain is malleable and ever-changing. These technologies have even helped researchers learn which parts of the brain are involved with different components of the memory process or with different types of memory. According to neuropsychologist and memory expert Larry Squire:

Memory appears to be stored as distributed ensembles of synaptic change. Neural networks are continuously resculpted as time passes after learning, i.e., there are both gains and losses of synaptic connectivity, and gradual changes in the substrate of memory. In general, what is understood about the biology of memory fits traditional psychological accounts of memory that emphasize its proneness to error and reconstruction, and change over time.[5]

Popular notions about memory have been challenged by scientific research. Just because someone is confident of her or his memory is by no means any guarantee that the memory is accurate; just because a memory is about a special, highly salient and meaningful experience, does not mean it is more accurate.

An example of how such popular notions are tested can be seen in a study by memory researchers Ulric Neisser and Nicole Harsch. The day after the explosion of the space shuttle Challenger, Neisser asked a group of students to write about how they first heard of the event. Three years later, the students were asked the same question again. They were also asked to rate how confident they were with the details of their memories, including where they were or who they were with. These answers were then compared to those from three years earlier.

After three years, those students who had shown a strong emotional reaction to the explosion by describing themselves as shocked, horrified or crying when the Challenger exploded, did not recall any better than the others. Although all the students remembered the explosion, they changed what they remembered, such as whether they learned about it from a friend or television. The researchers found that long-delayed recall even for "salient" events is often not accurate and confidence is not necessarily a reliable predictor of accuracy.[6]

Our memory works well for us. We usually remember our friends and colleagues, where the toothbrush is kept and when to pick up the dry cleaning. People seem especially good at remembering generalizations rather than all the tiny details. Our memories have succeeded in doing what is necessary for our civilization to have developed to where it is today. Our memories are wonderful and awesome and ever-changing. They do not, however, work like videotape recorders.

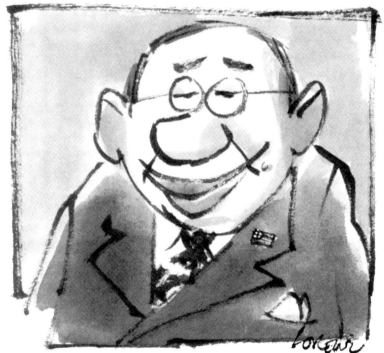

TODAY'S SPECIAL GUEST

BRUNDAGE MORNALD, OF
BATTLE CREEK, MONTANA

UNDER HYPNOSIS, MR. MORNALD
RECOVERED LONG-BURIED
MEMORIES OF A PERFECTLY
NORMAL, HAPPY CHILDHOOD.

Drawing by Lorenz; © 1993 The New Yorker Magazine, Inc.

When people think of hypnosis, they may conjure images of stage hypnotists levitating bodies or controlling people's actions. Hypnosis has been utilized as a part of sorcery, magic and medicine since ancient times. The scientific study of hypnosis began toward the end of the 18th century when a Viennese physician named Franz Anton Mesmer used it to treat patients. He called it "animal magnetism" in the mistaken belief that it was an occult force flowing through the hypnotist into the subject.

The study of "mesmerism" continued and came to be called "hypnosis" in the middle of the 19th century by English physician James Braid. Hypnosis was studied in both World Wars as a way to help soldiers who were victims of shell shock; it was recognized as a valid therapeutic practice in 1958. Hypnosis is often used to help control pain, for example. But is it good for retrieving memories? In 1992, hypnosis expert Michael Yapko asked about 1,000 practicing therapists for their views on hypnosis.

The following are three of the statements he presented. How would you respond?

(A) Agree Strongly (B) Agree Slightly
(C) Disagree Slightly   (D) Disagree Strongly

1. *Hypnotically obtained memories are more accurate than simply just remembering.*
    (A) (B) (C) (D)
2. *Hypnosis can be used to recover memories of actual events as far back as birth.*
    (A) (B) (C) (D)
3. *Therapists can have greater faith in details of a traumatic event when obtained hypnotically than otherwise.*
    (A) (B) (C) (D)

Yapko found that 43% agreed with the first statement, 54% agreed with the second and 47% agreed with the third.[1] When he published the results, alarm spread through much of the professional community.

75 percent of respondents thought of hypnosis as a tool for facilitating accurate recall whenever memories are otherwise not forthcoming.[2]

Why should we be alarmed? Because a

DILBERT

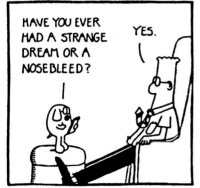

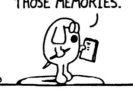

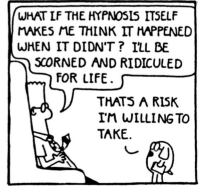

Doonesbury

BY GARRY TRUDEAU

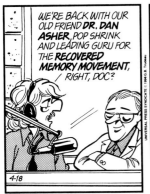
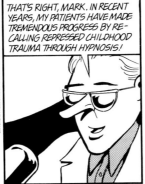
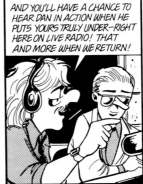
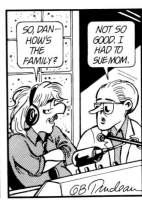

large body of research literature demonstrates that those therapists had mistaken beliefs about hypnosis.

Memories recovered through hypnosis are not more accurate than other memories.[3] While people may remember more details with hypnosis, they will also remember more inaccurate details despite feeling a heightened confidence about those memories. In fact, when a person agrees to undergo hypnosis, he or she is especially vulnerable to suggestion.

If memory worked like a videotape recorder, saving every image or experience, then it would be logical to use a tool such as hypnosis to find a particular saved segment. The therapists in Yapko's study who thought that people could remember events as far back as birth probably held this view of memory. But this is not the way memory works. We do not have a record of everything that we experience. Some information just does not get stored in our memory. Other information fades or gets lost.

Researchers have shown that adults do not maintain access to memories of events that happened when they were infants. This is referred to as the period of childhood amnesia and is a natural function of biological, conceptual and linguistic development. No process, no pill, no magic bullet can recover something that is not there to be gotten.

The therapists in Yapko's survey indicated that they had more faith in the details of traumatic memories that are recalled with hypnosis. While traumatic memories are generally more likely to be remembered, they are no less subject to change and reinterpretation than other memories. A recent study provides evidence for this.

Scientists examined 59 veterans of the Gulf War who were exposed to various traumatic war experiences. They interviewed the veterans soon after the experiences and recorded what the veterans told them about the events. Just two years later, they interviewed the veterans again. The scientists found that many of the reports of traumatic events had changed.[4] This is strong evidence that traumatic memories are subject to the same processes of change, decay and reinter-

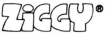

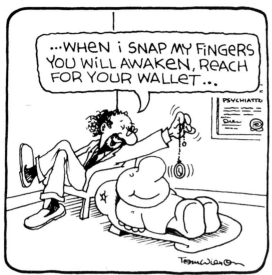

...WHEN i SNAP MY FiNGeRS YOU WiLL AWAKeN, ReACH FOR YOUR WALLeT...

pretation as other memories. Using hypnosis will not change the accuracy of the memory itself. If we want to be sure about the historical accuracy of the memory, we need to seek external corroboration.

Professionals have argued whether hypnosis is an altered mental state or whether it falls under a continuum of ordinary mental processes. Most would agree that:

Hypnosis involves the focusing of attention; increased responsiveness to suggestions; suspension of disbelief with a lowering of critical judgment; potential for altering perception, motor control, or memory in response to suggestions; and the subjective experience of responding involuntarily.[5]

Most people are familiar with "formal" hypnosis when patients are told that they are going to go into a "trance" state proceeded by a formal hypnotic induction. People are much less aware that hypnotic states can be achieved in an "informal" or "inadvertent" manner.

Many of the activities suggested by recovered memory therapists such as age regression, self-hypnosis, dream imagery, guided imagery, the use of sodium amytal, relaxation exercises or journaling can tap into the same uncritical mechanisms that underlie the experience of hypnosis.[6]

Despite the fact that there is no scientific evidence to support their beliefs, one study of Ph.D. psychologists indicated that 25% of the professionals who responded to the survey:

Believe that recovering memories is an important part of therapy, think they can identify clients with hidden memories during the initial session, and use two or more [hypnotic-like] techniques to help such clients recover suspected memories of CSA [child sexual abuse].[7]

In 1985, the American Medical Association warned:

Recollections obtained during hypnosis can involve confabulations and pseudomemories and not only fail to be more accurate, but actually appear to be less reliable than nonhypnotic recall.[8]

In 1993-1994, the AMA reaffirmed this statement noting that hypnosis and other memory-inducing techniques are "fraught with problems of potential misapplication."[9]

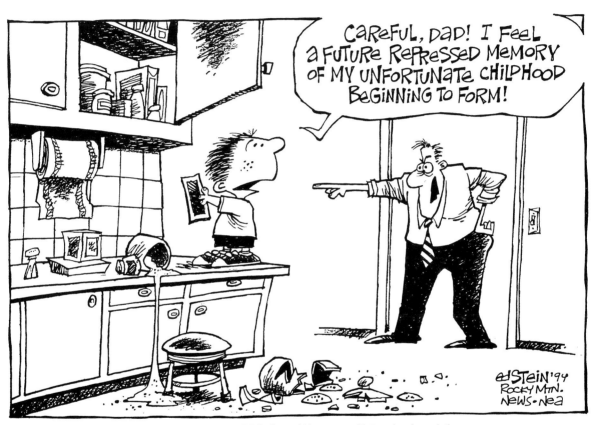

For most things in life it probably doesn't matter very much if we remember the precise truth or details of an event. Historical accuracy was not a major concern of therapy until recently and that concern is perhaps related to changes in the laws for reporting sexual abuse. Traditionally, therapists worked with what psychologist Donald Spence has called "narrative truth," the interpretation that patients gave to events in their lives to create an explanatory narrative.[1] Traditionally, the materials discussed by therapist and patient stayed within the confines of the therapy setting. That changed. Many therapists came to believe that their job was to validate their patients' recovered memories, even if they had no external corroboration, so great was the belief in the special accuracy of recovered traumatic memories.

Where did the idea that traumatic memories could be completely banished from consciousness and then be accurately retrieved come from? Psychiatrist Harrison Pope, Jr. looked to literature. He said, "If repression were a real phenomenon, experienced by human beings across the ages, we might reasonably expect to see it regularly in stories, poems, and dramas written throughout history."[2] He put the question to literary experts. No one in the Bible or in Shakespeare ever seemed to show a clear instance of repression. Nothing in classical Greek or Roman or Islamic literature was found. In fact, there was nothing in Western literature until the 19th century. Dr. Pope notes, "As best as we can tell, one of the first cases of repression and recovery of memory appears in James Fenimore Cooper's 1829 novel, *The Wept of Wish-Ton-Wish*,"[3] a tale in which children attacked by Indians repress and later recover memories. Pope notes, "Another possible case of repression arises in 1859, in Charles Dickens' novel, *A Tale of Two Cities*."[4] This is followed in 1862 with a reference by Emily Dickinson that an event could breed amnesia because it was too traumatic to contemplate. By 1896, with the publication of *Captains Courageous* by Rudyard Kipling, "repression and recovery of memory have entered romantic fiction in full-blown form."[5]

The notion of repres-

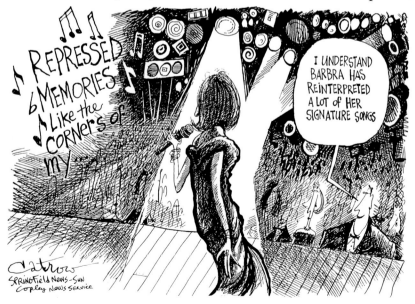

REPRESSED MEMORIES Like the CORNers of my...

I UNDERSTAND BARBRA HAS REINTERPRETED A LOT OF HER SIGNATURE SONGS

SPRINGFIELD NEWS-SUN
Copley News Service

sion, then, was already in the culture when Freud began his studies and developed his theories, which have had such a profound effect on American culture and psychotherapy. According to E. Fuller Torrey, a psychiatrist who is critical of much of Freudian theory, Freud:

> *Did believe that sexual abuse of children and sexual repression were the causes of anxiety neurosis, phobias, obsessions, [and] hysteria.* [6]

Freud is best known for his theories about the unconscious and the use of dreams although he did not invent the notion of the unconscious mind, which was commonplace in Europe prior to 1880. The techniques that he developed to reveal the repressions of childhood, however, are the basis of much of the recovered memory movement.[7]

The Freudian idea of a psychiatrist as an archaeologist who could uncover people's real memories was absorbed by our culture. The influence of movies carried the belief in childhood trauma and repression even further.

From the thrillers of Alfred Hitchcock to the

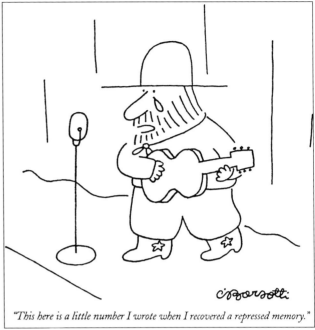

"This here is a little number I wrote when I recovered a repressed memory."

Drawing by C. Barsotti; © 1994 The New Yorker Magazine, Inc.

childhood trauma of Batman, characters in the movies regularly experience amnesia for traumatic events, and then, at some dramatic moment, recover the memory. Indeed, repression is the perfect device for Hollywood. Many a celluloid hero is seen having a "flashback"—a fleeting, freeze-frame image, perhaps slightly out of focus—of a long forgotten event.[8]

EEK & MEEK   **by Howle Schneider**

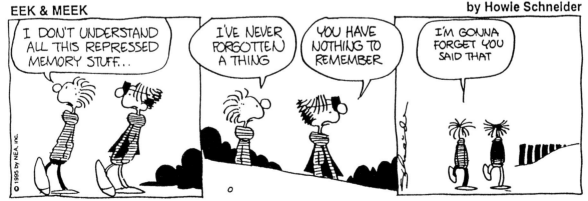

© 1995. Reprinted by permission of Newspaper Enterprise Association, Inc.

In America in the 20th century we have been surrounded by the notion of repression, so much so that it has come to seem real. It's been in our literature, our movies and professionally endorsed by psychiatry. What was forgotten is that "repression" was never more than an unsubstantiated theory. When critics began to question the reality of repressed memories, they questioned a cherished and long-held belief.

In 60 years of scientific research, however, no evidence has been found to support the reality of repression.[9] As the theory of repression has been questioned, those who believed in recovered memory therapy have changed. The terminology has replaced repression with dissociation.

Singer and Sincoff noted that repression is best conceptualized as "a pushing (or pulling) of ideas deep into the unconscious where they cannot be accessed"[10] and that dissociation is the "severing of the connections between various ideas and emotions."[11]

One of the scientists who has studied dissociative disorders in the laboratory says it seems unlikely that people would be symptom-free from the effects of traumatic stress for 20 or 30 years and suddenly start showing symptoms.

According to Harvard University psychology professor Daniel Schacter:

If people become skilled enough at dissociation to develop total amnesia for traumatic experiences, it would imply the existence of a dissociative disorder—a serious matter. If they have engaged in extensive dissociation, then patients who recover previously forgotten memories involving years of horrific abuse should also have a documented history of severe pathology that indicates a long-standing dissociative disorder.[12]

Whatever one calls it, there simply is a lack of evidence that people can accurately recall forgotten memories from the distant past. In the absence of external corroboration, we don't know if such long forgotten and then recalled memories are accurate or myths.

An accusation of sexual abuse creates a lasting stigma. In November 1995, *Dateline* asked 502 adults, "If someone has been charged and acquitted in a child abuse case, would you still be suspicious of them?" Poll results showed that 12% were not sure, 11% said no, that an acquittal would remove all suspicions and an overwhelming majority, 77% said yes, they would still be suspicious, even if the suspect was cleared.[13]

When a therapist makes a diagnosis of incest based on a "recovered memory," he or she gives an unfair sentence to the accused. When the topic is sexual abuse and the lives of many people are affected, it makes a great deal of difference whether a memory is a real memory or a myth.

Doonesbury

BY GARRY TRUDEAU

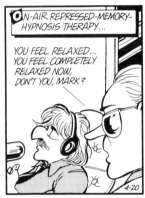
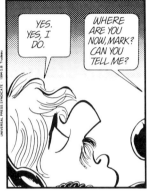
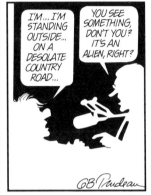
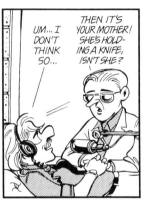
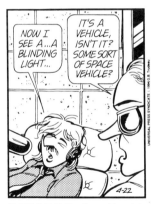
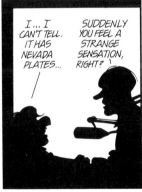
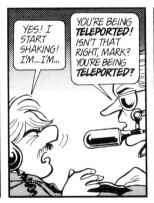
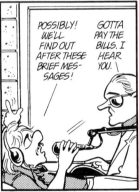

If people were not suggestible, there would be no need for advertisements. Large segments of our economy are based on the power of suggestion. From television commercials to free samples at the supermarket, to phone solicitation, who among us has not said "yes" when we really wanted to say "no" or made a purchase we really didn't want or need? How can we be convinced to buy things we didn't know we wanted or needed? It is because almost all of us succumb to the power of suggestion.

It seems ironic that suggestion is such an important component in our lives, but as a society, we seldom seem to take it into account—except in the advertising business. Psychologist Jonathan Schooler has noted:

A common error of the twentieth century has been the failure to appreciate just how susceptible individuals can be to the suggestions of individuals in positions of authority. Prior to World War II, few believed that people could be persuaded to carry out the atrocities that are known to have occurred.[1]

When Orson Welles did a broadcast of the Martian invasion, the public panicked. Who has not wondered how members of Heaven's Gate or Jonestown could have so willingly gone to their deaths? As Schooler remarks:

It seems there will always be people who can be convinced to believe just about anything. Why then should suggestions of prior sexual abuse be any different?[2]

What does this have to do with false memories?

Suggestion is inevitable within the context of psychotherapy—both direct and indirect. That seems obvious if one considers why someone goes to a therapist. People don't seek therapy when things are "going great." They go when they are having problems coping and are looking for help and guidance to change or improve their lives. When someone goes to a therapist, he or she has sought out an expert, someone who has special knowledge or talents. An expert is usually someone

Well, there has to be a reason your life is screwed up! Were you abused as a child?

If you say so!

Dr. Shrink

Gamble © 1994, The Florida Times-Union.

40

Kudzu

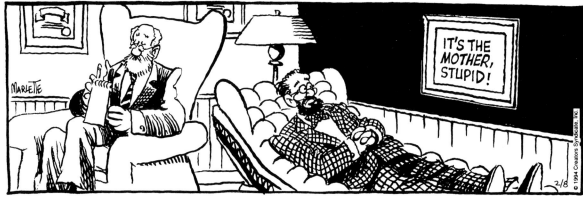

who receives payment for service. And patients usually follow an expert's advice in order to relieve their painful symptoms and get better. There is nothing wrong with this as long as everyone involved is aware that this is the context of therapy.

Memory researcher Martin Conway, states: *Indeed, experimentally inducing false memories in healthy young adults appears almost trivially easy, the implication being that in the context of therapy, with a patient who is psychologically dysfunctional and actively seeking help, the probability of memory distortion and fabrication is multiplied many times over.*[3]

Psychologist and hypnosis expert Michael Yapko, has remarked:

One need not question whether someone is suggestible, but instead assess the degree of suggestibility at a given point in time or in a given context. One need not employ formal hypnotic or suggestive techniques for the purpose of recovering presumably repressed memories in order to impart the assumption that such memories exist and the expectation that such memories can

and will be found.[4]

The notion that patients become absorbed in their therapists belief systems is not a new one. It was known decades ago that patients who went to Freudian therapists had "Freudian dreams" and those who went to Jungian therapists had "Jungian dreams." But can people be led to believe that they were abused when, in fact, they never were? Yapko notes:

Case examples of virtually impossible forms of abuse that are vividly "remembered" make it clear that the answer is yes.[5]

Memory researchers have proven that certain factors may increase suggestibility. For example, asking someone to imagine that something happened can be a highly suggestive process because imagination and memory can be confused. In addition, imagining events can make a person feel more confident that the events actually occurred. Imagining events also increases the chance of producing a false recollection.[6]

When a therapist, Renee Fredrickson for example, suggests to her patients that for six months they imagine they had been abused, she is using a risky technique because it increases the chance for false memories to develop. When people are asked about things repeatedly, it increases the chance for suggestion,[7] and when they are placed in groups whose members all claim a belief in something, people seem to conform to the group.[8] And yet, therapy techniques for recovering memories do just this. The techniques that have been used to recover memories of sexual abuse are techniques that incorporate great potential for suggestion. Cognitive psychologists agree with the following statement by Schooler:

> The use of memory recovery techniques for the specific purpose of recovering memories of sexual abuse that are unbeknownst to the patient seems quite *dangerous indeed!*[9]

When therapists recommend sexual abuse literature or participation in a survivor group to patients who have no memory of being abused, it clearly communicates to the patients that the therapist suspects abuse occured, planting a powerful suggestion from a trusted authority.

Actually participating in a survivor group or reading sexual abuse books provides patients with the necessary knowledge regarding the sexual abuse "scripts." In short, while such suggestive techniques might sometimes aid in the recovery of long-lost memories, "they represent the very type of procedure that cognitive psychologists would likely recommend if one explicitly wanted to plant a false memory of abuse."[10]

Committed By Michael Fry

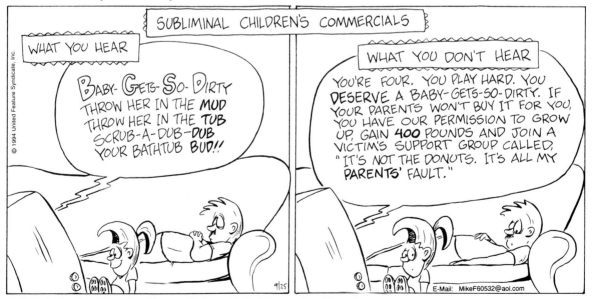

LAWTON
USA

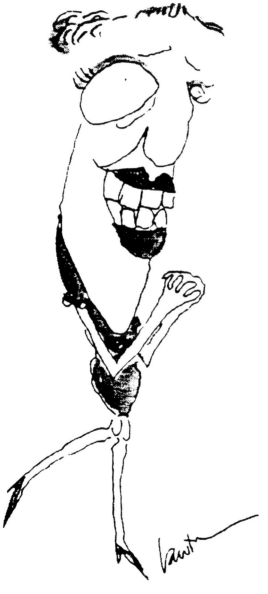

In 1995, Margaret Singer and Janja Lalich published a book entitled *"Crazy" Therapies.* In it they documented many of the seemingly crazy things that people have tried in an effort to ease their angst or find self-fulfillment or meaning in their lives. From primal screams to hot tubs, no idea seems too far-fetched to try.[1]

A peek into any New Age magazine reveals therapists offering help through crystals, chanting, channeling, aromatherapy, therapeutic touching, electromagnetic fields and wagging a finger before a patient's eyes. There are literally hundreds of therapies available but only behavioral and cognitive therapies have been demonstrated to be effective through scientific evaluation.

The type of crazy therapy that is most related to the recovered repressed memory movement is regression therapy. Can we really go back and re-experience our childhood, our birth or a past life? The premise of age regression hypnosis techniques is "yes" we can. The evaluation of scientific researchers is "no" we can't.

Hypnosis is the basis of age regression. After being hypnotized, a patient is directed to move backward in time to a specific period; and then, with the guidance of the therapist, re-experience memories from that time. Individuals in regressed states can seem very convincing, often demonstrating a great deal of emotion, they may even seem to talk and behave like a young child. The experience of age regression can be so vivid and intense that the hypnotized person may come to believe the elicited "memories" actually happened.

Most schools of psychotherapy assume that childhood experiences form an adult's personality. Some therapists assume that they can actually regress their patients to childhood. These therapists believe that through "rebirthing" or "reparenting" the mistakes made by the parents will be uncovered, that they must be confronted and then the patient will be understood.

By the late 1940s some therapists were proclaiming that their patients' parents were unloving, mean, intrusive, and

Calvin and Hobbes   by Bill Watterson

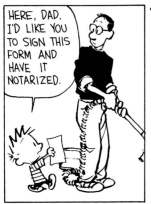
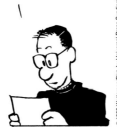
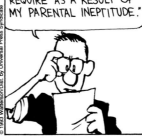
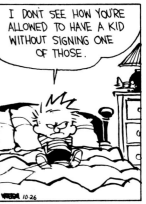

Ick

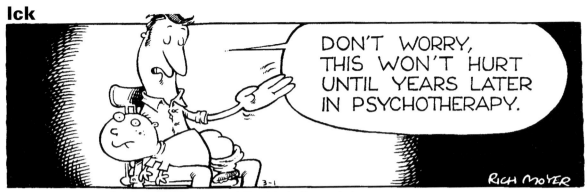

DON'T WORRY, THIS WON'T HURT UNTIL YEARS LATER IN PSYCHOTHERAPY.

RICH MOYER

controlling, and had in effect harmed, if not ruined, their offspring. From there, some therapists deduced the solution that the all-loving therapist would restore the patients by bringing them up properly.[2]

Age regression continues to be popular, especially in New Age circles. Brian Weiss, a Yale University educated psychiatrist, has a waiting list of thousands who are willing to pay huge amounts of money to be regressed to past lives.

Promoted uncritically by talk shows where the concern is for ratings and not the well-being of participants or viewers, past life regressions have been performed on *Donahue, Oprah, Joan Rivers, Montel Williams,* as well as on CNN. Celebrity entertainer Shirley MacLaine has been promoting age regression and other New Age beliefs for many years.

Space alien abduction therapy received much publicity after Harvard professor John Mack added to its credibility with his publication of *Abduction: Human Encounters with Aliens*, which is also based on regression techniques.[3] Although it has been thoroughly debunked, its adherents still flock to meetings, and were it not dangerous, we could laugh at regression therapy. Unfortunately, it can be dangerous.

No one monitors hypnotherapists. There

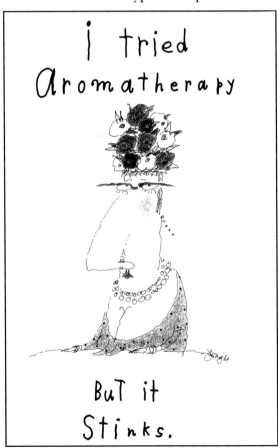

i tried aromatherapy

but it stinks.

are no prerequisites for training. There are no licenses. There is no organization to which hypnotherapists are accountable. Anyone can attend a weekend seminar and obtain a piece of paper to hang on the wall asserting that he or she is a "certified hypnotherapist."

A well publicized example of the harm that can be done by regression therapy was the 1991 suicide of Paul Lozano, a medical student who was the first patient to be age regressed by Harvard psychiatrist Margaret Bean-Bayog. Dr. Bean-Bayog regressed Lozano to age three and then suggested that she would be his mother, concluding that Lozano had been sexually abused by his own mother. Dr. Bayog sent him children's books as gifts and wrote notes to him referring to herself as his "mom." After the suicide, Lozano's family received a settlement from a lawsuit they had filed. Court records in the lawsuit revealed that other professionals who saw Lozano felt the treatment he received was harmful.[4]

It is difficult to understand why regression therapy is tolerated. As long ago as 1985, the American Medical Association warned of the dangers of confabulation with the use of hypnosis.[5] In 1987, memory researcher Michael Nash published a review of the available research on age regression showing that claims of accurate recall, actual thinking like a child and perceiving like a child did not hold up under scrutiny.[6]

The drawings of people who were regressed to childhood, for example, have been found to be more mature than drawings of actual children of that age.

Even though hypnotically regressed subjects may undergo dramatic changes in their behavior and feelings, their performance is not accurately childlike. People who are hypnotized and told to progress to age 70 or 80 give equally compelling portrayals. Hypnotic age regression may elicit a profoundly believed-in experience, "but it does not seem to involve a bonafide return to or reinstatement of childhood functioning."[7]

NON SEQUITUR

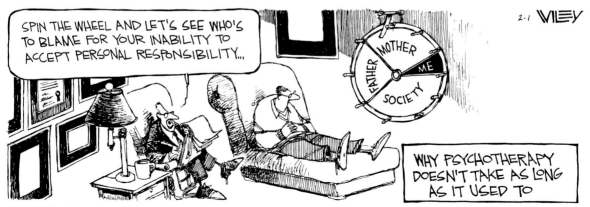

SPIN THE WHEEL AND LET'S SEE WHO'S TO BLAME FOR YOUR INABILITY TO ACCEPT PERSONAL RESPONSIBILITY...

FATHER MOTHER ME SOCIETY

2·1 WILEY

WHY PSYCHOTHERAPY DOESN'T TAKE AS LONG AS IT USED TO

© 1994, Washington Post Writers Group. Reprinted with permission.

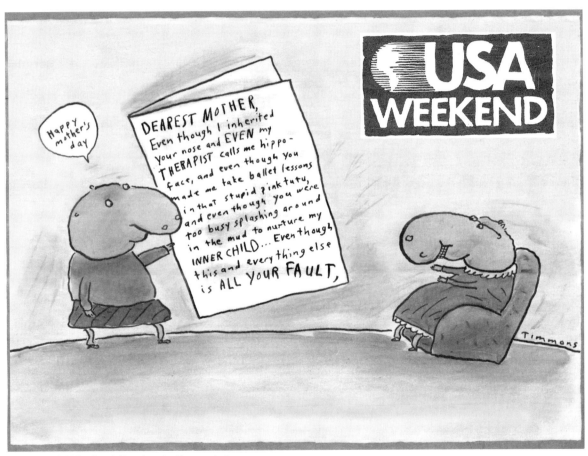

© 1992, USA Weekend. Reprinted with permission.

In 1969, Canadian therapist and addiction researcher/social worker, Margaret Cork, presented the first modern study on children of alcoholic parents in "The Forgotten Children." According to Cork, adult "children of alcoholics sustain lasting psychological damage."[1]

In 1977, a small group of Al-Anon members (Friends and Family of Alcoholics) gathered in New York City for the first meeting of adult children of alcoholics. In the late 1970s, a New Jersey based therapist, Janet Geringer-Woititz, began working with a group of adults who had been raised in alcoholic households. She later published *Adult Children of Alcoholics,* which reached *The New York Times* best seller list. It was said that Dr. Woititz's study and resulting book "broke new ground in our understanding what it is to be an Adult Child of an Alcoholic."[2] The book has since been translated into German, French, Norwegian and Polish. But has it really broken new ground and uncovered the "inner child?"

As a result of international exposure, an increasing number of people today are calling themselves "adult children." The self-help book market as well as national media exposure have helped promote this concept.

The "adult child" movement grew out of the belief that children of alcoholic families are neglected, physically and/or sexually abused, sensitized to drug and/or alcohol use in the family, deprived of love and attention, or overindulged and grow up suppressing explosive amounts of anger. The metaphor inner child is used in popular literature for coping with these emotions. The inner child "protects" the abused child

HOWARD HUGE

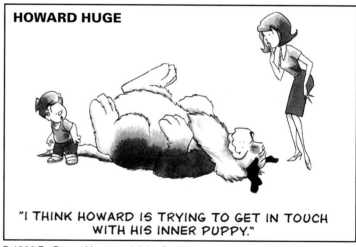

"I THINK HOWARD IS TRYING TO GET IN TOUCH WITH HIS INNER PUPPY."

DAVE

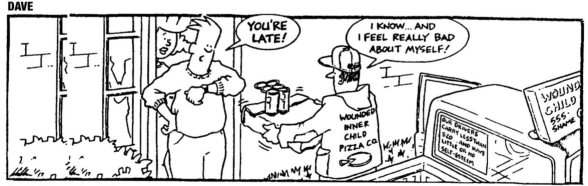

MOTHER GOOSE & GRIMM

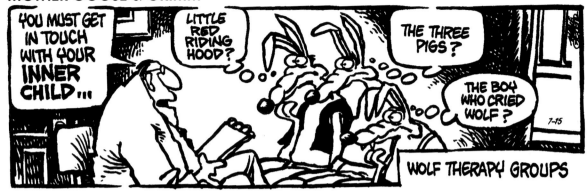

by placing or forming memory blocks, locking away these traumatic experiences. When the abused child reaches adulthood, these blocked and unresolved issues are believed to surface and create problems. According to the Adult Children Educational Foundation, an adult child is "trapped in the fears and reactions of a

Child, and the Child who was forced to be an Adult without going through the natural stages that would result in a healthy Adult."[3]

John Bradshaw has helped promulgate these ideas. In fact, he suggests:

The crisis is not just about how we raise our children; it's about a hundred million people who look like adults, talk and dress like adults, but actually are adult children.[4]

Who or what is the inner child? The

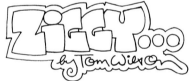

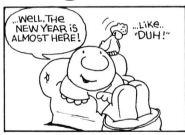

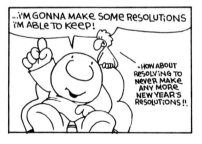

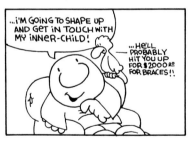

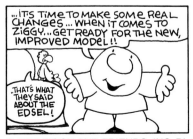

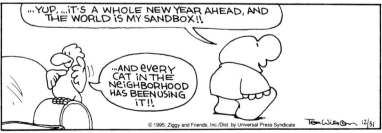

inner child is in effect the abused child's protector. The inner child supposedly harbors forgotten memories of abuse. Recovery therapists recommend that people treat their inner child (a symbolic reference perhaps for inner strength and/or courage) as a very real, living, breathing child who needs love, attention and cuddling. They say you have to:

Earn the respect of your Inner Child. . . . When you approach the Inner Child, you will usually find that memories will return.[5]

Some therapists encourage their clients to hug and cuddle either a teddy bear or a soft pillow and address it as an independent identity, for example:

Laugh Parade

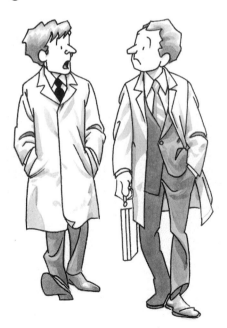

"I FREED MY INNER CHILD, AND NOW HE WON'T LET ME PLAY WITH HIS TOYS."

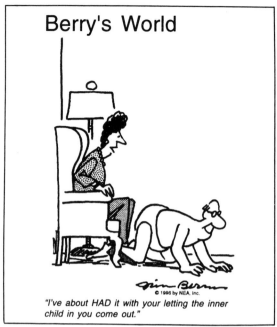

Berry's World

"I've about HAD it with your letting the inner child in you come out."

Client: I love you (tears), you're a good boy and you deserve to be loved even if you make a mess. You deserve to have someone to love you and play with you.

Therapist: Now each day you can spend a few minutes with your little child letting him know that he is loved and cared for.[6]

Although the inner child is a metaphor for people in recovery, the inner child assumes a new meaning and becomes real in the minds of so-called survivors. Inner children even converse on the internet.

In 1993, in his book *The Invisible Wound*, therapist Wayne Kritsberg presented diagrams locating one's inner child. "The picture locates the inner child in the lower belly area, where the body stores most of the pain of sexual abuse."[7]

The inner child metaphor has been carried to the extreme.

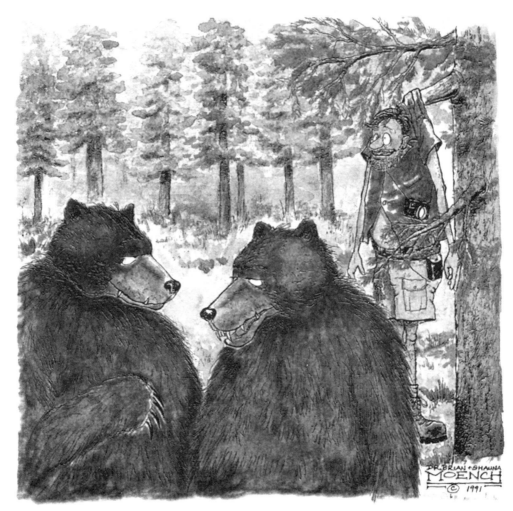

"His name's Bradshaw. He says he understands I came from a single parent den with inadequate role models. He senses that my dysfunctional behavior is shame based and codependent and he urges me to let my inner cub heal .... I say we eat him."

He has been called the world's greatest communicator. He has written five books which have all reached *The New York Times* best seller list. He is the creator and host of four nationally broadcast PBS television series. He has been nominated for an Emmy Award for Best Talk/Service Host. He presents lectures and workshops around the country, filling convention halls and auditoriums with as many as 7,000 people at a time. He has appeared on *Oprah*, *Donahue* and *Geraldo*. Barbra Streisand and Nick Nolte are among his good friends.

On the other hand, John Bradshaw is considered by thousands to be a sham; a person whose preaching has destroyed countless families. His message is: We are all part of the patriarchy; the patriarchy is responsible for creating dysfunctional families; often we must reparent our inner child and we must break with our dysfunc-

tional "family of origin" and find a new, healthy "family of choice."

More than anyone else, Bradshaw is responsible for pioneering the concept of the "wounded inner child." He has helped create hundreds of thousands of adult children, who spend an inordinate amount of time searching for perpetrators and accusing their parents, grandparents, siblings and countless others of destroying their lives. The theory suggests that virtually everyone was wounded in child-hood, and in order to become healthy adults we must heal our inner child. Of course, the inner child is only a metaphor, but to Bradshaw followers the inner child is a living, breathing, vulnerable person.

Bradshaw preaches that parents were often the abusers. Bradshaw's idea of a dysfunctional family is one that is tradition-ally patriarchal, rules by fear and "promotes the denial of feelings and corporal punish-

THE DUPLEX   BY GLENN MCCOY

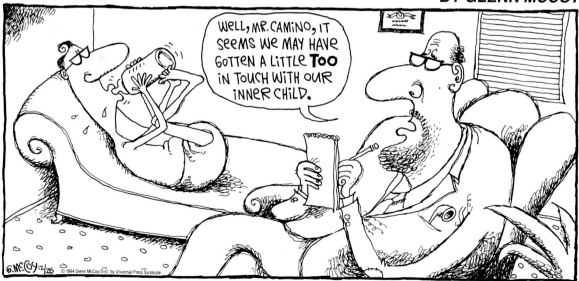

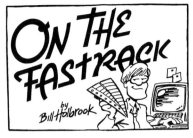
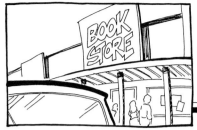
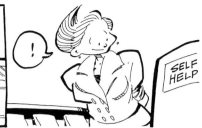
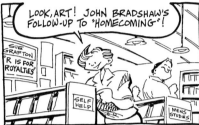
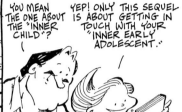
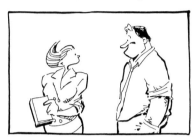
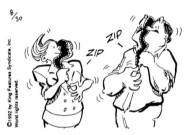
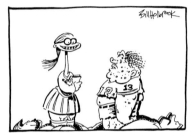
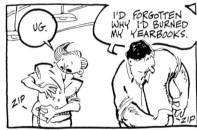

ment."[1] In the late 1980s and into the 1990s, tens of thousands of parents who thought they were good parents raising happy, well-adjusted children, suddenly found themselves accused of being child abusers. Some fathers, who at first encouraged their adult children to attend John Bradshaw workshops, later discovered that the child returning from this seminar was full of hatred, callously casting accusations, breaking from his or her family, and sometimes even pursuing the family in court. The workshops encourage the wounded adult child to regress to childhood, find that wounded inner child and recover memories of supposedly long-forgotten abuse.

Bradshaw's first book, *Bradshaw On: The Family*, was published in 1988. The book was immensely successful. In fact, it served as the impetus for the first PBS series, also titled *Bradshaw On: The Family*. The following are some of the notions it espouses. On the dysfunctional family in crisis, he comments:

[Hitler] used the socialization structures of the German family to create the Nazi regime. As long as the poisonous pedagogy goes unchallenged, the phenomenon of Hitler is still a potential in our society.[2]

And again when profiling a dysfunctional family, Bradshaw notes:

Nonfunctional families are shame-based. . . . the rules are rigid and unchang-

53

ing. The poisonous pedagogy helps to set up these rules. The dominant rules are control, perfectionism, blame.[3]

John Bradshaw has convinced tens of thousands of people that their failed interpersonal relationships—food, sex, alcohol, drug addictions, depression, phobias, and all sorts of disorders and dysfunctions—are "shame-based syndromes."[4] A former preacher, Bradshaw's message is that a higher power can help you recover "to get back to healthy shame."[5] When asked whether that higher power, that unattainable spirituality must be God, Bradshaw replies:

> *You can recover without believing in God. . . . Higher power can be the group or the therapist. You have to think this person or this group knows more than "I" do.*[6]

When people wonder why intelligent sons and daughters would accept a therapist's treatment that is so destructive, they should understand that "trust" is the underlying concept in therapy. A person is continuously reminded that healing can take place only if one yields power and trusts a higher power. That higher power can be the therapist. Vulnerable people are susceptible to control and manipulation.

In his workshops, Bradshaw uses mind-altering techniques such as imaging and visualization. This is what he says about original justice work:

> *It's very very scary work, but for a lot of people who have been severely violated, they'll need to do it. It's a re-enactment of abuse, it involves heavy grief work. When a little girl is being violated sexually, she wants to scream, cry, and hit back, but she*

Farcus

by David Waisglass
Gordon Coulthart

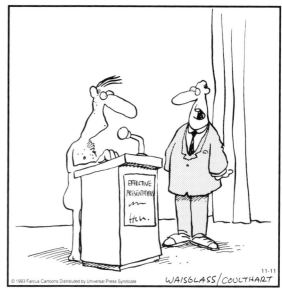

© 1993 Farcus Cartoons Distributed by Universal Press Syndicate WAISGLASS/COULTHART

"It seems you misunderstood when I said you should visualize the audience naked."

> *can't. She has frozen energy, and that energy has to be completed. It's also called original vindication work.*
>
> *Clients picture their offender's face and beat it with a bataka stick. Some people say it promotes violence but I say it's what will prevent violence. A lot of treatment centers fear this work, it's very powerful—there's trembling, sobbing, primitive guttural sounds, but for some it's necessary. It's the legitimate suffering Jung talks about. It's like a vindication and restores the person to [a] sense of dignity.*[7]

These techniques, which are similar to hypnosis, should also be used cautiously. Is Bradshaw so naive that he does not understand the powerful suggestibility in such an activity?

Doonesbury G.B. Trudeau

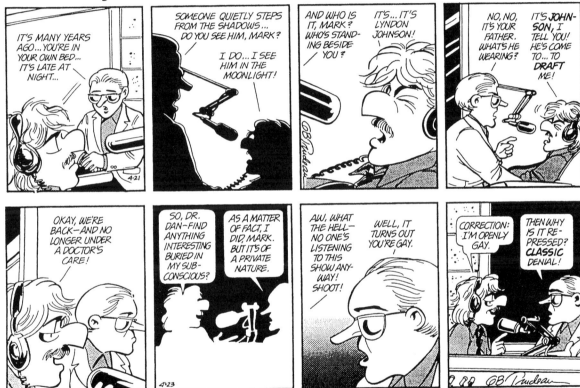

Accused: "I didn't do it!"
Accuser: "Perpetrators always deny their guilt and that is evidence that you are guilty."

How can you deal with this circular logic? According to the above scenario, if an accused person admits to committing the crime, then he or she is guilty. But if the accused person denies the crime, the same conclusion is drawn–*guilty*. This is not logical thinking and doesn't allow the accused to present a defense.

What is even more troubling is where the patient retracts a "memory" and is told he or she is in denial and that is proof of abuse. It is like the witch trials at Salem, where women were thrown into ponds. If they floated they were guilty and burned, if they sank they were innocent—but dead. It is a no-win situation.[1]

In 1994, a woman described her experience to the False Memory Syndrome Foundation: She was arrested for drunk driving. "I was guilty of the charge," she explained:

But what happened during the interview was so strange that I wanted you to know. The officer who interviewed me had a check list of items: age, address and so forth. But then he asked a series of "yes" and "no" type questions such as, "Have you ever been arrested before?" One of the questions asked if I had been abused. To all of these questions I answered "No," but the manner in which my

answers were recorded was quite interesting. Although [the officer] wrote "no" next to the question about the past arrests, he wrote "denies abuse" next to the question about whether I had been abused in the past.[2]

In other words, if you have never forgotten your abuse, then you were abused. If you have no memory of being abused, then you are "in denial".

How did this circular reasoning develop and enter the mainstream? The term, in denial, was first used in alcohol treatment programs such as Alcoholics Anonymous (AA). In fact, in denial is a concept in the first step of AA's 12-Step Program: "We

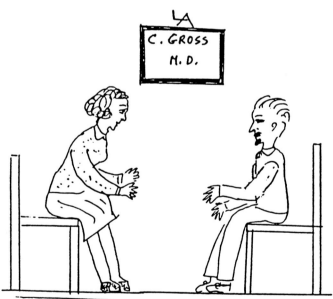

"But Doc, I don't think that one of my personalities is a prostitute." "Hon you are in denial. Just count your money in the evening and in the morning, and you will see that I am right."

(This is a true story as reported by a recanter in Canada.)
Reprinted courtesy of Paula Tyroler.

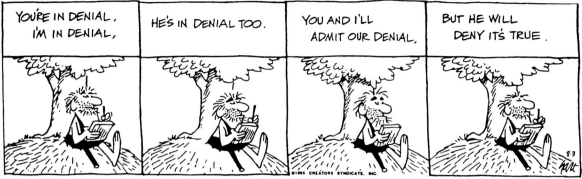

YOU'RE IN DENIAL, I'M IN DENIAL,

HE'S IN DENIAL TOO.

YOU AND I'LL ADMIT OUR DENIAL,

BUT HE WILL DENY IT'S TRUE.

admitted we were powerless over alcohol—that our lives had become unmanageable."[3] Simply put, in order to begin treatment, the alcoholic must first recognize and admit that he or she has a problem—an alcoholic must first overcome his or her denial of the problem.

This idea has been so widely communicated that many people have come to accept it and believe it to be true. Furthermore, AA doctrine warns that practicing alcoholics live in a continuous state of denial, unwilling to accept their condition or their dependency. AA's *Big Book* states that an alcoholic is capable of recovery, and that "he can only be defeated by an attitude of intolerance or belligerent denial."[4] Alcoholics who refuse to acknowledge their alcoholism are said to be in denial. Critics point out that "portions of the recovery movement have created a catch-22 situation. Since denial is a symptom of alcoholism, then if you deny being an alcoholic, that proves that you are one."[5]

It is claimed that our society is in deep denial—not only about alcohol and drug abuse, but also about such issues as child abuse and incest. One recovery movement promoter has said that "wherever there's denial, secrets, control, there's addiction."[6] Denial is fundamental to the dogma of Alcoholics Anonymous, and it has now become fundamental to the recovery movement.

In the early 1980s, the AA movement became a model for other groups.

According to British scholar Richard Webster:

One of the crucial factors associated with the rise of the recovered memory movement was the extensive denial of the reality of child sexual abuse. The denial of the experience of women and children who genuinely had been victims of sexual abuse provided the essential conditions without which the recovered memory movement could never have grown and flourished the way that it did.[7]

Pop psychology and self-help books state, "Denial gives you a respite when you cannot bear to align yourself with that small, wounded child for another minute. . . . It is a survival skill."[8] And recovery guru John Bradshaw advised his followers, "The first step in recovery is to break down these denials and go find what

Maybe that "normal, happy childhood" you think you had wasn't so normal and happy after all.

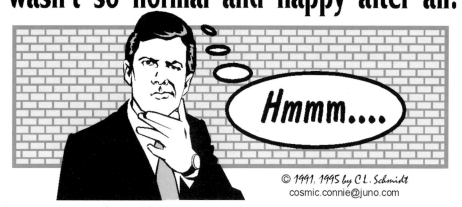

Hmmm....

© 1991, 1995 by C.L. Schmidt
cosmic.connie@juno.com

Isn't it time you considered a career as an Incest Survivor?

I call a family of choice."[9]

When patients question the veracity of their recovered memories of childhood abuse, they are said to be in denial. In the words of one recovered memory therapist: "Following the memory, there's almost always denial. 'I don't believe this; this didn't happen.' "[10]

At each successive session, the patient is reassured that his or her denial is a symptom of the abuse, and that he or she will never get better unless the denying stops and the memories are accepted as truth. Clients are not simply encouraged to believe that they were abused, but pressured to accept the abuse diagnosis. Those "bold enough to reject the diagnosis of incest survivor [are] said to be 'in denial,' unwilling to confront the truth; the rejection of the diagnosis is *prima facie* evidence in its favor."[11] Essentially, "if the client admits the abuse happened, it happened; if the client doesn't admit it happened, it *still* happened."[12]

Even retractors, people who have said the memories they developed in therapy were wrong, have been branded as being in denial. "Why should we believe the memories of retractors? They are just denying the abuse again."[13]

Patients are in a "no-win" situation and are ultimately victimized by their therapists. They are admonished to accept their symptoms as "the foreordained 'truth' of their abuse."[14] It is the patients who are the victims—suspended between trusting his or her therapist's wisdom and trusting their own gut instincts.

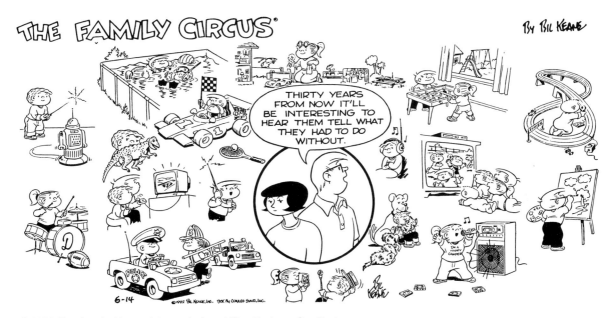

© 1992. Reprinted with special permission of King Features Syndicate.

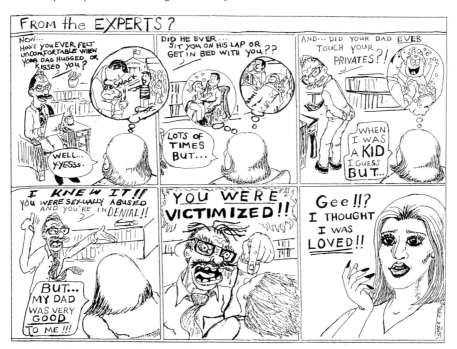

Reprinted with permission of Sharon Gornic.

They were called baby boomers and the me-generation. They were the most cared-for generation of children in the nation's history. Post World War II babies, they grew up in boom times. Many of their fathers were former G.I.s. Their parents were well educated, optimistic and energetic. They grew up in the tumultuous sixties, when idealism abounded, and in the seventies and eighties, when prosperity provided them with luxury not seen before in this country or anywhere else in the world.

But in the 1980s and 1990s, something went wrong. Unaccustomed to adversity, many members of this generation began to consider themselves as victims. They began to call themselves adult children and attend self-help groups in droves. The expectations for these children were great. With all the advantages they had, they expected perfection and happiness, which their parents could not provide. Disappointed, they looked for answers to their discontent. Misguided, perhaps well-meaning counse-

QUALITY TIME   Gail Machlis

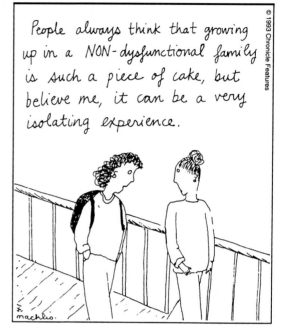

lors told them in their self-help groups and seminars, and in hundreds of books, that any disappointments in life were not their doing, but likely were attributed to parenting mishaps.

It became common in therapy circles to

Calvin and Hobbes   by Bill Watterson

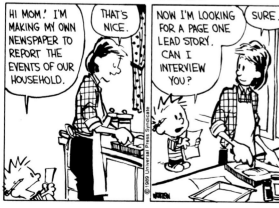
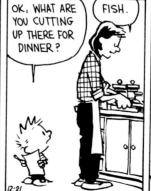
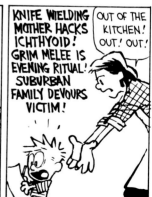

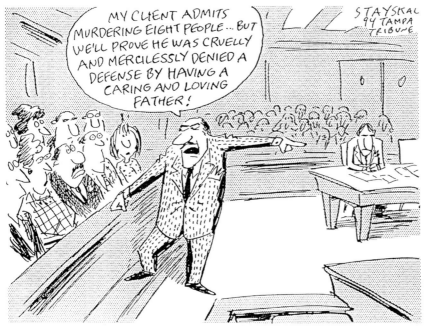

© 1994. Reprinted courtesy of Wayne Stayskal.

QUALITY TIME   Gail Machlis

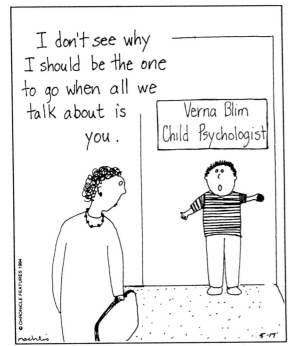

© 1994 Gail Machlis. Reprinted courtesy of Chronicle
Features, San Francisco, California. All rights reserved.

proclaim that the only way to healing was to delve into the past, locate and confront the perpetrators and separate from them, not speaking with anyone who disagreed with the interpretations of new-found memories and emerging accusations.

Tens of thousands of parents who had devoted their lives to their children were dumbfounded. Their children were sitting in judgment and would not give parents a chance to respond.

The amazing aspect of this phenomenon is that it hit the most unlikely cohort of citizens. Strong, caring, loving, successful families were under attack everywhere in the nation and other English-speaking countries as well.

The False Memory Syndrome Foundation (FMSF) was founded in 1992 to seek answers to this phenomenon. In 1993, the FMS Foundation published the results of a Family Survey.[1] This is what they found from about 500 families who responded:

71% of mothers were at home with children

71% of families are active in churches

71% of parents are still married

These statistics are above average for the

typical American family. Most of these mothers were there when their children arrived home from school; they were there to help with homework and drive carpools; they were able to take the time to prepare the family meal that the family generally ate together. Both parents attended PTA and parent-teacher meetings and took an active interest, often volunteering numerous hours in their children's school and extracurricular activities. These familial units were strong, with family gatherings, vacations and church get-togethers. Compared to today's statistics, the divorce rate was significantly lower.

In these families, 70% of the siblings do not believe the accusations. Almost 30% of the

Berry's World

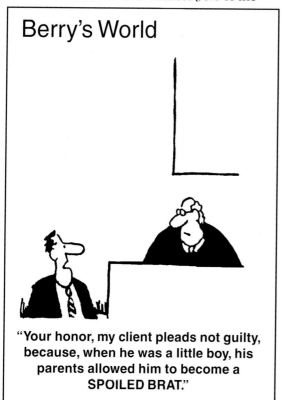

"Your honor, my client pleads not guilty, because, when he was a little boy, his parents allowed him to become a SPOILED BRAT."

Bizarro — by Dan Piraro

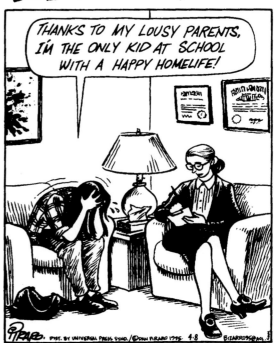

accusing women have post-college education.

The survey indicated that for the most part these families lived lives that were considered exemplary for their times. They showered their children with affection and attention.

This information raises a profound philosophical question: Are so-called good parents bad for you? Do such parents make life too easy, too comfortable? Is a child in such a family left with too little challenge? Do seemingly good families provide too much love and shelter, which in turn, does not provide the child a realistic view of the world?

The truly abused child may have excuses for problems in life. Is the abuse excuse so acceptable that it has been pre-empted by others to find answers for the disappointments in their lives?

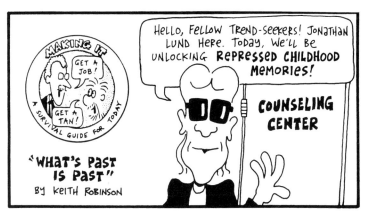

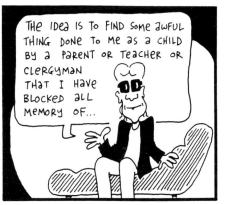

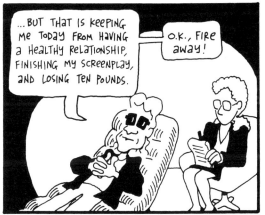

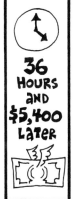

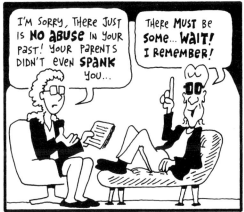

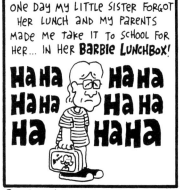

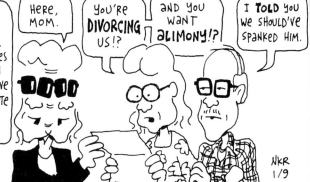

Reprinted with permission of Making It Productions, www.makingit.com

At this time I don't feel that I can see you or Dad, or have you visit us at home. . . . I am making my healing a priority in my life now.

My responsibility is to resolve my pain and in order to do that I need no contact with you.

Until I get a clearer picture of who did this to me, I wish to have no contact with either of you.

I am writing to say good-bye to you. It's been a year now since you and I last met and, Dad, it's apparent after this much time just how unwilling you are to be reconciled with me. . . . If you desire reconciliation, please do as I have asked you in the past—see a therapist.[1]

Among the many aspects of the recovered memory and false memory phenomenon, the most disturbing behavior to parents has been the "cutting off" or severing of contact by their accusing adult children. The comments above are from some of the thousands of letters received by parents and forwarded to the FMS Foundation.

Cutting-off seems to have become part of the recommended behavior for someone who claims to be a "survivor." Parents are devastated by this behavior because they fear that they have lost their child and can no longer reason with him or her. "Isolation" and cutting off contact are the very same techniques utilized by cults to control information and prevent exposure to alternative ideas. Cutting off contact from any person who does not agree with one's beliefs is cult-like behavior.

Isolation is not a new idea in psychiatry. In *A History of Psychiatry,* Edward Shorter, an anthropologist who studies the history of medicine, reminds us that as early as 1817, there was the recommendation that "removal from family and friends would contribute greatly to diverting the patient from the previously unhealthy persons that had ruled his or her life."[2] Shorter also writes that "the notion of isolating asylum patients from friends and family was also very familiar. Historically, these are techniques that each generation of psychiatrists invents for itself."[3]

The current practice of

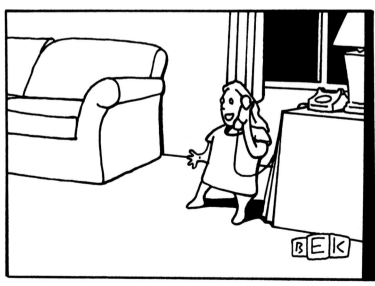

"So, are you still with the same parents?"

detachment from the family appears to be a merger of ideas from the branch of psychiatry that considered it necessary for the therapist to "reparent" a patient with ideas from alcohol recovery programs. In the 1940s and 1950s, untold thousands of mothers were labeled "schizophreno-genic" and were considered to be the cause of their children's schizophrenia. Some therapists viewed their job as "reparenting" the children. The alcohol recovery idea is described by a Pennsylvania therapy group called Genesis. The Genesis approach, according to their statements, attempts to parallel the Alcoholics Anonymous model.

It has long been accepted in Alcoholics Anonymous (AA) that an individual will likely not stay sober while being around addictive, unhealthy "persons, places and things." As a parallel philosophy, we firmly believe that while a client is working through ACOA issues in therapy and making the transition from dysfunctional to healthy, it is necessary to detach from the dysfunctional environment.[4]

Cutting off is not a matter of choice: it is required.

Detachment is never easy, but it must be done to accomplish two of the goals of therapy: to reparent the child within and to mourn a lost childhood. . . . We require our clients to detach from their caregivers of origin during the therapeutic process.[5]

The idea that, in order to heal, a patient must leave her "family of origin" and join a "family of choice" permeates the survivor literature. Indeed, cutting off from family seems to be part of the expected role for a survivor. Beverly Engle tells readers that "permanent separation is usually the only possible resolution if either parent . . . either directly or indirectly brings you only pain when you get together."[6] Engle provides explicit instructions on how to divorce your parents.

You may decide to divorce your parents in person. In this case, refer to the confrontation preparation exercise described earlier. If you have been able to successfully complete this exercise, you are probably ready for a real face-to-face good-bye. As you did in the exercise, choose a safe place for your meeting. Know what you are going to say ahead of time, and make sure you say everything you want to say. There is no need for discussion; just say your good-byes, and leave.[7]

John Briere, Ph.D. and professor at the School of Medicine of the University of Southern California, spoke of "parent-ectomy" and "psychological surgery" when suggesting that cutting off is warranted if the "nonoffending" parent directly or consciously defends the molester and negates the survivor.[8]

Christine Courtois, clinical director for the Center of Abuse Recovery and Empowerment at the Psychiatric Institute of Washington, writes:

Survivors must also decide how to interact with their families of origin—whether to maintain full or limited contact or to "divorce" themselves from the family. Limited contact or total estrangement often leads a survivor to "refamily" with her partner and children or to find a

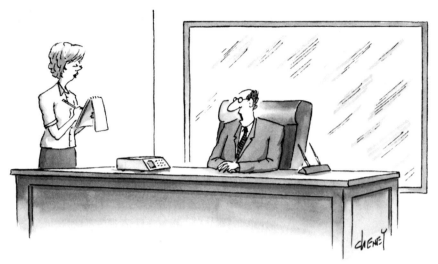

" 'You pushy, manipulative, tyrannical scum . . .' Scratch that. 'Dear Mom and Dad . . .' "

because the perpetrator could hang up the telephone. If the confrontation is to be in person, then it is generally recommended that it be held in the therapist's office and highly orchestrated and rehearsed.

Ellen Bass and Laura Davis tell survivors:

The initial confrontation is not the time to discuss the issues, to listen to your abuser's side of the story, or to wait around to deal with everyone's reactions. Go in, say what you need to say, and get out. Make it quick. If you want to have a dialogue, do it another time.[10]

Renee Fredrickson in *Repressed Memories: A Journey to Recovery From Sexual Abuse*, recommends:

Avoid being tentative about your repressed memories. Do not just tell them; express them as truth. If months or years down the road, you find you are mistaken about details, you can always apologize and set the record straight. . . . You cannot wait until you are doubt-free to disclose to your family. This may never happen.[11]

"Confrontation with alleged perpetrators solely for the supposed curative effect of expressing anger should not be encouraged. There is no reliable evidence that such actions are therapeutic."[12]

surrogate family, people with whom she can develop family bonds and traditions and with whom she can celebrate special occasions and holidays.[9]

Hand in hand with cutting off from the family of origin is the notion of confrontation. It is the nature of the confrontations that prompted families to call them "hit-and-run" accusations. Although conceived as a way to empower survivors, the confrontations seem more like ambushes to families. Survivors are told that by confronting their abusers they regain their power, but they are warned that the "perpetrator" will deny the abuse. There are a number of things that are recommended so that survivors can keep control of the situation. Sometimes the survivor has a ceremonial confrontation that does not involve the perpetrator. This can be play-acted with a survivor group. If the perpetrator is to be involved in the confrontation, then writing a letter is considered better than a phone call

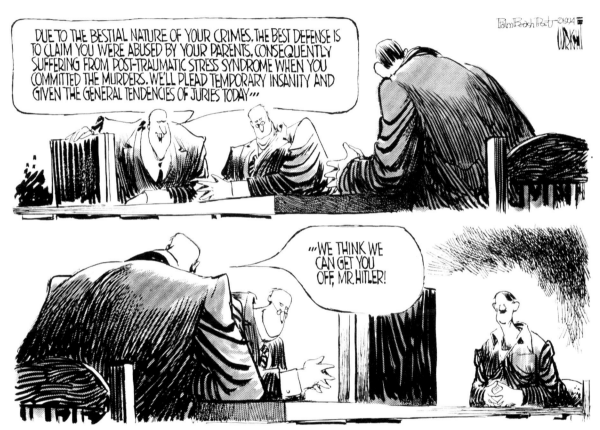

Reprinted with permission from Don Wright, THE PALM BEACH POST.

The Post-traumatic Stress Disorder (PTSD) diagnosis was introduced into the *Diagnostic and Statistical Manual of Mental Disorders (DSM III)* in 1980 as a way to account for some of the late developing symptoms of Vietnam combat veterans. The ailment had previously been known as "combat fatigue syndrome," which referred to people who were rendered nervous at the time of some terrible event and who continued to suffer over time. The PTSD diagnosis required that a patient must have experienced a trauma outside the range of normal human experience and that the trauma would have been distressful to almost anyone who experienced it.[1]

Over time, the criteria for this diagnosis changed. Many clinicians ignored the 1980 requirement and extended the PTSD diagnosis to include negative events within "normal human experience."

For example, feminist psychologists argued that all women suffer from PTSD by nature of living in a patriarchal society.[2] A reflection of the broader criteria is apparent in the 1994 edition of the *DSM IV*, in which the diagnosis of PTSD was changed

to include almost any experience that was severely frightening.

The PTSD diagnosis is closely related to the recovered memory issue. The memory of the trauma may have a delayed onset. Delayed onset was interpreted not in terms of days, weeks, months or even years but in decades. The evidence that there had been a trauma was based on symptoms. The trauma was inferred. The diagnosis acquired a one-size-fits-all character.

The idea that a person might not remember being sexually abused is recent. Before introducing a woman who claimed that she had recovered her memories from many

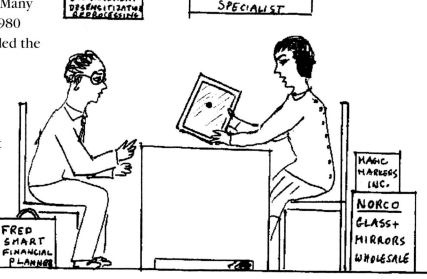

"Fred, I discovered new therapy for PTSD called MA-EMDR Mirror-assisted EMDR, which the patients can do at home. They make a dot on a mirror, look at it, and move their head from side to side."
"Amazing, Dr. Biway! But how are you going to make money?"
"Simple! I'll be selling mirrors and magic markers, and I'll train therapists how to train their patients."

Reprinted with permission from Paula Tyroler.

TANK McNAMARA®   by Jeff Millar & Bill Hinds

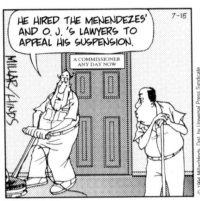
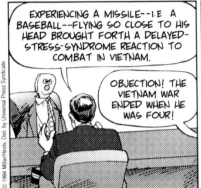
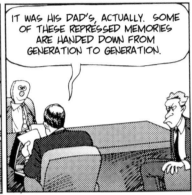

years ago, Oprah (January 17, 1991) demonstrated this change with the following comment:

> It's an incredible thing because, you know, when I first used to read about cases like this, I, thinking I'm halfway intelligent, would say, "How could a person not remember." I mean, if you were sexually abused, how could you not remember that. And I say that because I was and I do remember. [3]

Many professionals are uncomfortable with the new PTSD diagnosis. Some have expressed concern that the symptoms of PTSD described by recovered memory therapists are a result of the therapy rather than occuring prior to therapy. For example, medical records of some former patients show that they did not have PTSD symptoms until they started recovering memories.[4]

Another concern of some professionals is that the symptoms of PTSD are similar to those of long established mood and anxiety disorders and they question the need for this additional category. Others argue that

PTSD is unlike the other entries in the *DSM* because PTSD requires a causal agent (trauma) for a diagnosis. And still others are uncomfortable because a diagnosis of PTSD seems to reflect a physician's personal style more than it does a specific ailment.

If a therapist diagnoses PTSD in a patient who has no memories of a trauma, the therapist is likely to urge the patient to uncover the memories of the trauma. This tends to be long-term therapy. Physicians who use the traditional categories indicated by the patient's symptoms are more likely to treat and alleviate those symptoms. This tends to be short-term therapy.

PTSD has influenced social views. Vietnam veterans who had previously been treated as social outcasts were transformed into victims with the introduction of the 1980 diagnosis. "Men and women who had been scorned became eligible for disability benefits and improved mental health services."[5] Indeed, a PTSD diagnosis also has "marketing appeal" because it doesn't have the stigma possessed by other psychiatric disorders. As one PTSD proponent wrote:

PTSD is an attractive explanatory model for many people because it places responsibility for their suffering on factors outside themselves, factors over which they often had neither responsibility nor control.[6]

The PTSD diagnosis had a profound impact on the law. It "offers the law a scientific rationale to support the socio-political ideology of victimization and to justify the growing recognition of victims' rights."[7]

It has been invoked as a defense in a number of different crimes. "PTSD is almost unique in its capacity to convey to jurors both a 'scientific' explanation of the defendant's nonresponsibility and a sympathetic account of his victim status mitigating his blameworthiness."[8] The conceptual leap in the law regarding the effects of the PTSD diagnosis are represented in cases covering a range of issues from automobile accidents to battered woman syndrome, rape trauma syndrome, victims' rights and victims' compensation, and both intentional and negligent infliction of emotional distress.

One can actually see the PTSD diagnosis evolving and encompassing even more situations. First, the definition of PTSD included the necessity of experiencing a trauma beyond the normal life experience; it then expanded to include experiencing anything negative. Now, it seems that PTSD has become contagious with those at greatest risk of catching it, being therapists who listen to the stories of their clients. An increasing number of professional articles and research studies are examining what has come to be referred to as "vicarious traumatization." A therapist training video called "Vicarious Traumatization" informs therapists about "the cumulative impact of trauma clients' stories and reenactments."[9] And notes that "the bottom line is that working with trauma survivors changes us profoundly."[10]

Even children are now at risk for catching PTSD. According to the Sidron Foundation, a group that vigorously supports recovered memory therapy, "children can be vicariously traumatized by living with a dissociative parent who may be self-destructive or prone to flashbacks of trauma experiences."[11]

As these changes occur, we might ask if we are turning ordinary life events into mental illness. Is the grief that follows the death of a loved one a pathology or a normal life experience, for example? Some see professional responses to death and disaster as the growth area for the psychologist and counselor industry.[12] And families have complained that professionals did not allow them to deal privately with their grief.

We are not expected to be capable of handling trauma—a word surrounded by the sound of its own importance, a word few knew a half-century ago—or almost any emotional state, even positive ones, alone....We need professionals.... Do we, though?[13]

Regardless of one's feelings concerning the PTSD diagnosis and the sociopolitical changes it has reflected or inspired, Posttraumatic Stress Disorder is the medical foundation on which a culture of victimization has been constructed.

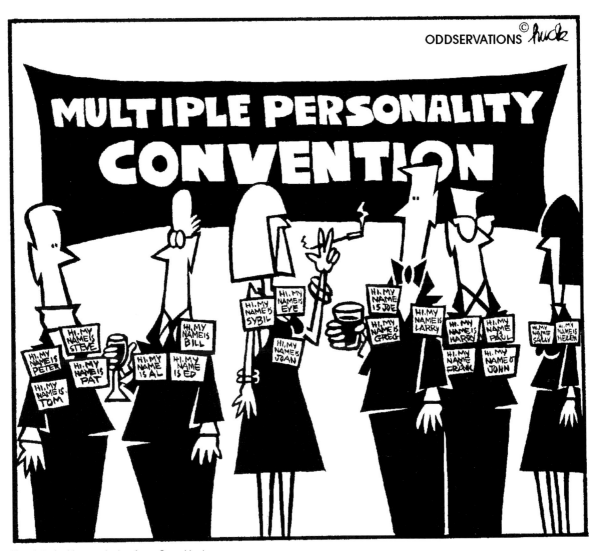

Reprinted with permission from Gary Huck.

The diagnosis of Multiple Personality Disorder (MPD) has sharply divided the medical community. In 1994, the name was changed to Dissociative Identity Disorder (DID), although many still refer to it as MPD. Some believe MPD is common in our society, affecting at least 1% of the population,[1] while others believe it is an artifact of the therapy process and a result of the techniques used by therapists.[2]

Before 1980, there were about 200 people in recorded history throughout the world in whom this disorder had been diagnosed.[3] In 1980, MPD was entered into the *Diagnostic and Statistical Manual (DSM III)*. Since then, many agree it has been widely overdiagnosed. A senior vice president of the mental health arm of Aetna states that there are 10 times as many Multiple Personality Disorder claims as there were 10 years ago.[4]

MPD is said to be "characterized by the presence of 'alter personalities' that periodically and unpredictably take control of the patient's body."[5] By doing so, these "guest personalities" cause out-of-character behavior for which the "host personality" often claims amnesia. Unfortunately, the notion of "personality" is poorly defined. Thus, no definition or set of criteria exists to determine whether or not a particular set of behaviors is due to an "alter" personality.

There are no behaviors that are exclusive to MPD. For example, symptoms of "anxiety disorders, psychoses, various personality disorders, schizophrenia, somatization disorder, affective disorders, alcoholic 'blackouts,' various kinds of substance abuse, seizures, eating disorders, any medical condition"[6] could all be viewed as the behaviors of alter personalities. According to psychiatrist August Piper, there is no way to correctly verify that a diagnosis is MPD and not some other diagnosis. Nor is there any way to prove that a person does not have MPD.

In other words, the diagnosis is not falsifiable. That means it fails to meet a fundamental tenet of science: it cannot be shown to be false.

An additional problem of the MPD diagnosis is that there is no way to distinguish between lying or malingering behavior. Indeed, it is "quite easy for behavior characteristic of different personalities to be role-played or induced, with or without hypnosis."[7]

The behaviors associated with MPD have

MISTER BOFFO
by Joe Martin

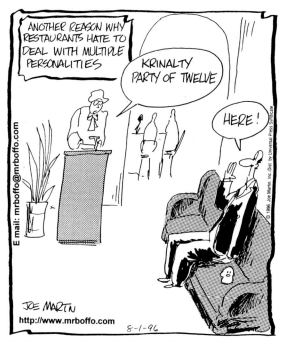

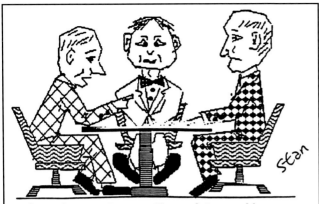

I get three votes; my therapist says I have Multiple Personality Disorder.

Reprinted courtesy of Stan Stevens.

been observed in other cultures and time periods, sometimes called "demonic possession."[8] In the late 19th century, French psychologist Dr. Pierre Janet and Boston neuropsychiatrist Morton Prince "proposed that a psychiatric illness involving multiple personalities existed."[9] Interest in this diagnosis waned, however, until the late 1950s and early 1960s when the book and later the movie, *The Three Faces of Eve*, burst upon our culture.

MPD critics have pointed out that the supposed cause of MPD changed as books appeared in popular literature. It was only after the publication in 1973 of Cornelia Wilbur's *Sybil*, for example, that childhood physical and sexual abuse were "widely recognized as precipitants of multiple personality."[10]

In addition to changed beliefs about the causes of MPD, the number of "alters" diagnosed in patients also changed. Although the first cases noted two or three

personalities, by the late 1980s we find reports of 300 to 4,500 personalities[11] and even alters who claimed to be cows or dogs or ducks.

The authors of *The Three Faces of Eve* considered MPD a rare condition. Herbert Spiegel, M.D., who also treated Sybil, did not agree with therapist Cornelia Wilbur that Sybil was a Multiple Personality.[12] Despite the critics and the warnings by those who brought MPD back into public awareness, the diagnosis continues to have great popularity. Perhaps the diagnosis of MPD is appealing to patients because they are told that they have a special talent for surviving difficult experiences. It is not unusual to see references from patients who refer to their "gift" of being multiple.[13]

Another appeal may be that the diagnosis removes their responsibility for their symptoms and problems. They can blame their problems on someone else.

"What happens to the concept of responsibility in a society were scores of thousands

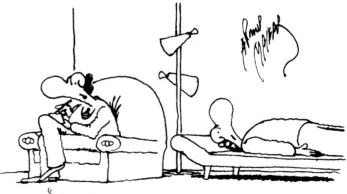

"MULTIPLE PERSONALITIES IS SUCH A COLD TERM, MR FLAGG. LET'S JUST SAY YOU HAVE A SWISS ARMY LIFE."

Reprinted courtesy of Scott Masear.

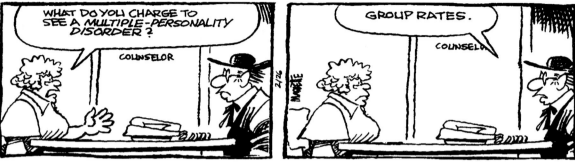

of people receive this diagnosis?"[14] It is this aspect of multiple personality disorder that has made many ordinary people question the diagnosis because it conflicts with our traditional culture and legal system. MPD is a peculiarly American disease and is seldom diagnosed in other countries.[15] It seems that some people have used MPD to avoid taking responsibility for their actions. Headlines such as the following have become all too common:

Accused Blames Mental Disorder: Embezzlement Suspect Claims to Have Multiple Personalities[16]

Judge Told Woman's Child Self Was Thief[17]

How do the claims of MPD patients, who say that they didn't know what their alters were doing, differ from the claims of those seeking to avoid taking responsibility for their actions? No one knows.

In addition to all these problems, treatment for MPD is also expensive. Therapy may last anywhere from three to over five years and often includes frequent and long hospitilization.[18]

In 1984, Martin Orne and his colleagues suggested criteria for the diagnosis of MPD. Perhaps their application could help resolve the problems with this diagnosis. According to Orne, a diagnosis of MPD should meet at least the following criteria:

1) There should be evidence that the condition existed before contact with the clinician who makes the diagnosis.
2) The various personalities should be consistent over time.
3) The personalities should not be readily changed by social cues.[19]

Until the therapy community dispels doubts about the MPD diagnosis, public concern that MPD is a product of therapy will likely increase. The headline below is indicative of the problem that exists:

Doctor Accused of Bogus Therapy, Bills Appleton Woman Says Former Psychiatrist Convinced Her of Many Personalities, Billed for Group Therapy [20]

Such headlines may make people snicker.

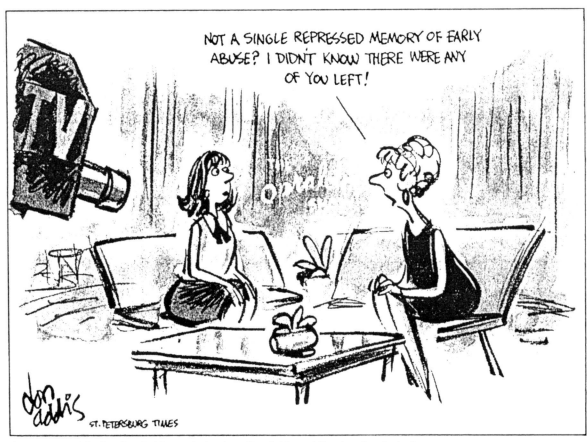

© 1994 Don Addis. Reprinted with permission from Don Addis and Creators Syndicate, Inc.

For entertainment during the 18th century, Britishers could traipse to the asylum of St. Mary of Bethlehem where (for a fee) they could gawk at the insane people who were on display. The word "bedlam" entered our language from the popular pronunciation of the name of that infamous place. Most of us like to think that as a society we have progressed and that our attitudes and treatment of the mentally ill are more humane.

Where might we look to see what attitudes are reflected in our culture? Virtually every home in the country has television. In half a century, television has become the dominant influence on the opinions and lives of people. As the influence of television has grown, the distinction between news and entertainment has blurred. Nowhere is this clearer than in the daytime talk shows of people such as Oprah Winfrey, Phil Donahue, Geraldo, Leeza and Ricki Lake. In 1995, about 150 daytime talk shows were available to viewers on a weekly basis.[1]

Driven by ratings, these programs vied to attract viewers by offering the most outrageous, bizarre, sickest and weirdest people they could find. Sensationalism sells. There seems to be no end and no limit to the public disclosures of private matters that talk show hosts will air.

Daytime talk shows have been a highly significant factor in spreading misinformation concerning memory and mental health. Hosts who give their "unconditional positive regard" to a presidential candidate on Tuesday may give the same unconditional positive regard on Wednesday to someone who claims to have been sexually abused by aliens on board a spaceship. Unconditional positive regard may arguably be a good therapy concept, but it makes for confusing journalism. For the viewer, it makes distinguishing fact from fantasy much more difficult.

Talk show hosts are authority figures. They have a huge following, sometimes with as many as 20 million viewers. In November 1992, 1/3 of the people in the country who were watching television were tuned in to *Oprah*.[2]

An example of how the false memory

One Big Happy

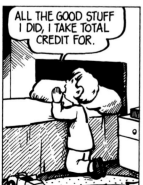 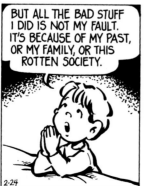 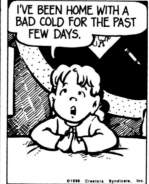 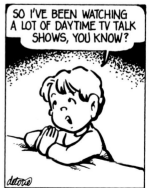

© 1996. Reprinted with permission from Creators Syndicate, Inc.

problem was propelled by talk show hosts can be drawn from Roseanne Barr's announcement that she was an incest survivor to a group in a Denver church on September 21, 1991. A media frenzy followed. On *Sally Jessy Raphael* (October 10, 1991), Roseanne said: "I remember my mother molesting me while she was changing my diaper."[3] What might have happened if rather than giving unconditional positive regard, Sally had asked Roseanne: "What about childhood amnesia and the fact that there is no evidence that people can remember events from such a young age?" Instead, Sally gave Roseanne the talk-show-seal-of-approval, saying:

I have been greatly moved by what I believe is a great deal of courage to speak out. . . . So if you are saying to me, 'What do you think? What do you feel? Do you believe her?' The answer is, darn right, I do.[4]

And just a month later on *Oprah* (November 8, 1991), Roseanne said: "When someone asks you, 'Were you sexually abused as a child?' There's only two answers. One of them is, 'Yes,' and one of them is, 'I don't know.'"[5] What would have happened if instead of giving unconditional positive regard, Oprah had pointed out the absurdity of that statement—or at the very least its political implications?

Roseanne went on to claim that she had

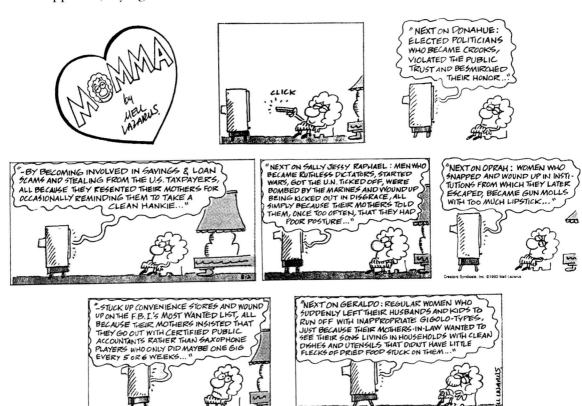

© 1992 Mell Lazarus. Reprinted with permission from Mell Lazarus and Creators Syndicate, Inc.

also developed 21 multiple personalities, instantly becoming the
ultimate marketing tool for a
mental illness.[6] On a *Leeza* show,
Roseanne described her disorder:
"It's a gift that allows you to be
multiply gifted."[7] What would
have happened if Leeza had
asked: "What about the
conflict within the psychiatric profession over this
diagnosis?" Or, "what
about the excruciating
histories people diag-
nosed with MPD have
endured?"

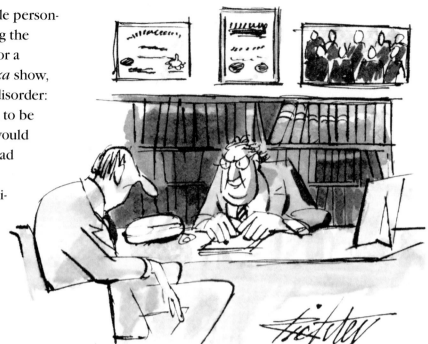

*"Your case has been turned down by Oprah, but we're
appealing to Sally Jessy Raphael."*

Drawing by Richter; © 1995 The New Yorker Magazine, Inc.

Television talk shows
have made a parody of
mental health treatment
by exploiting people's
intimate problems and
portraying them as
entertainment. Sometimes it seems that we
have not come so very far from bedlam
after all.

Television has been a moving force in the
spread of the incorrect notions of the recovered memory movement, but it is also a
powerful force in bringing the movement to
an end. While some of the television news
journals and movies gave credibility to
notions of recovered repressed memories,
MPD and satanic ritual abuse by their uncritical acceptance of claims, some of these same
programs have now started to reflect the
mounting skepticism.

False memory syndrome has been the
topic of a soap opera series, of many news

reports and of an extensive *Frontline*
documentary, "Divided Memories."[8] Television news journals and talk shows have
presented reports of the experiences of
families, of retractors, and recently, of
lawsuits. Special reports have explained
the constructive nature of memory and the
power of suggestion.

In fact, through the media, the country
has had an ongoing course in recent devel-
opments in memory research. As solid
scientific information continues to be aired
and as the public is exposed to skepticism,
people will be in a better position to make
informed decisions about the recovered
memory movement.

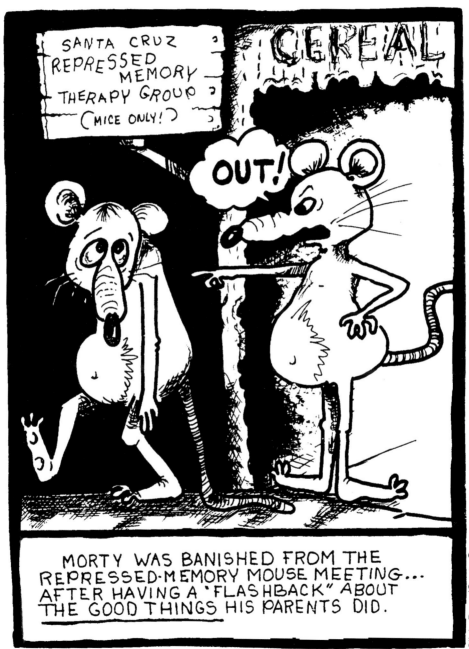

Reprinted with permission from the Santa Cruz County Sentinel.

Most people take at least three to five years of working a fairly intense recovery program.[1]

Recovery from incest is a long-term, ongoing process.[2]

I'm going to need therapy for the rest of my life.[3]

Alcoholics Anonymous' (AA) 12-Step program was adopted as a model for incest recovery programs. In AA, members often speak of "working the program" meaning that they work through each of the 12 Steps toward recovery from alcoholism. Admitting that you are powerless in the face of alcohol and making amends to people who have been harmed are two steps, for example.[4] In the context of the "incest recovery movement," however, "working the program" takes participants on a contorted journey into the beliefs and technologies of New Age as a way to uncover "memories" and feelings.

REMEMBERING INCEST & CHILDHOOD ABUSE IS THE FIRST STEP TO HEALING. WE CAN HELP YOU REMEMBER & HEAL[5]

This was the message on an advertisement from one treatment center. The ad also included a list of symptoms that could indicate whether the reader might need the help of this center. With irritable bowel and migraine headaches on the list—who would not qualify!

The same treatment center listed the components of its program: "Inner Child, Self Parenting, Rage Work, Psychodrama, Body Work, Memory Recall, Narco Analysis, Exercise, Play Therapy."[6] Other techniques that are often included in incest recovery programs are: dream work, group work, feelings work, guided imagery work, hypnosis, family of origin work, journal and confrontation work.

Dream Work is done in the belief that dreams and nightmares represent explicit accounts of sexual abuse that took place during childhood. Therapists utilize a variety of methods to do dream work. For example, dream work therapist Carol Conger:

Often has her workshop participants use Tarot cards in dream work. The dreamer draws a Tarot card to represent the significant symbols and characters in her dream. She then associates to the symbolism of the

SHOE

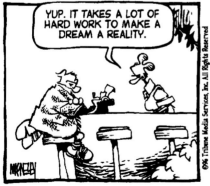
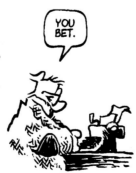
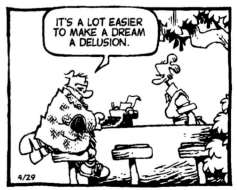

Tarot card as a pathway to a deeper understanding of the symbolism of her dream.[7]

Is dream work a reliable way to recover accurate memories? The answer is no, there is no reliable evidence that dreams represent historically accurate memories.

Body Work is based on an unfounded belief that "though the mind may repress or deny the reality of the abuse, the body always stores the memory and gives the greatest testimony to its occurrence . . . the body never forgets."[8] The theory that "the body stores the memories of incest"[9] has been widespread. Massage therapy is probably the most common body work technique, but cranio-sacral therapy, polarity therapy (deep relaxation), reflexology, rolfing, soma (realign muscles and bones), dance, exercise and aerobics are also used to help "recover memories."[10]

Group Work: According to therapist Mike Lew, group work can be a powerful means of helping a person take charge of his or her life.

It is impossible to overstress the benefits of being able to share your feelings and experiences with other incest survivors. There is no more powerful contradiction to isolation than telling your story to people who . . . believe you.[11]

A group is supposed to provide a safe haven where speakers are given unconditional belief and support. Survivors are encouraged to "tell your story again and again"[12] because that makes the story become more real. "As the story is repeated, more details are recovered."[13] The problems with this are obvious:

as stories are repeated, people naturally embellish and they also pick up details and ideas from other people's stories. In addition, research has shown that repeating a story helps it to become more firmly believed—whether accurate or inaccurate.

Rage Work has its origins in the belief that people need to express their anger in order to be healthy. Investigative reporter Debbie Nathan attended a retreat for survivors that included rage work. Of the approximately three dozen women attending the retreat, eleven had no memories. Nathan wrote:

On each mattress was a telephone book. "Pretend the phone books are your perpetrators," Beth instructed us. "Get mad at them. Beat the fuckers with the hoses. Scream! Scream as loud as you can! Hit as hard as you can! Challenge yourself to get angry. Then your inner children will take over. Your rage will come. Your healing. And your memories."[14]

Typically in such sessions, participants without memories are asked to imagine someone who might be the perpetrator and use his name. Most participants continue to hold much anger for the person whom they imagined they were hitting with the hoses.[15]

Memory Work: When survivors are embarked on a journey of memory work, they feel that they have reached a landmark if they have a *flashback*. "Flashbacks are unbidden, often vivid, images (or a sequence of images) that occur while the patient is awake."[16] The word, flashback, has been used synonymously for "memory" in the survivor literature although there is no evidence that flashbacks necessarily

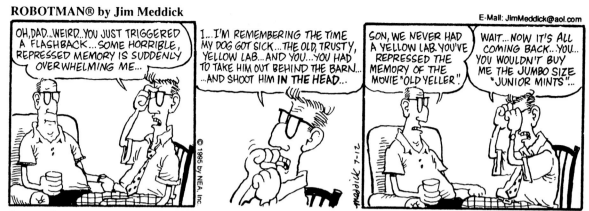

ROBOTMAN® by Jim Meddick   E-Mail: JimMeddick@aol.com

Panel 1: OH, DAD...WEIRD...YOU JUST TRIGGERED A FLASHBACK...SOME HORRIBLE, REPRESSED MEMORY IS SUDDENLY OVERWHELMING ME...

Panel 2: I...I'M REMEMBERING THE TIME MY DOG GOT SICK...THE OLD, TRUSTY, YELLOW LAB...AND YOU...YOU HAD TO TAKE HIM OUT BEHIND THE BARN......AND SHOOT HIM **IN THE HEAD**...

Panel 3: SON, WE NEVER HAD A YELLOW LAB. YOU'VE REPRESSED THE MEMORY OF THE MOVIE "OLD YELLER".

Panel 4: WAIT...NOW IT'S ALL COMING BACK...YOU...YOU WOULDN'T BUY ME THE JUMBO SIZE "JUNIOR MINTS"...

represent historically accurate memories.

The term, flashback, was coined to describe the visual images of people who were taking hallucinogenic drugs. According to some professionals, flashbacks represent a worst case scenario. For example, a person who had a minor fender-bender in the afternoon might have a flashback later in the evening in which the car is demolished. Like dreams, flashbacks can have their source in imagination and the only way to know if they are historically accurate is to find external corroboration.

Many therapists use "guided imagery" to help clients recover memories, not realizing that this is a hypnotic-like process. In guided imagery, clients are asked to imagine places and events suggested by the therapist. Some therapists are very direct and suggest that their patients imagine what it was like to be abused. "Spend time imagining that you were sexually abused, without worrying about accuracy, proving anything, or having your ideas make sense."[17] Research has shown that the simple act of imagining an event can lead many people to actually believe that the event took place.[18]

The use of photographs to help uncover memories is very common. Psychologist John Briere describes this technique:

Many photographs of incest victims and their families superficially suggest happiness and togetherness—all members may be smiling and apparently enjoying themselves. With closer examination, the rigidity of this posture becomes apparent, and the "happy family" facade may seem almost garish or surreal.[19]

With Briere, if people in a family photo look unhappy they must be unhappy. If they look happy they must also be unhappy. No family can withstand such undermining.

Survival work is mostly about finding memories. It is based on the incorrect assumption that if someone can find the right playback button, he or she can replay an actual event. There is simply no scientific support that any of the memory work techniques can do that. Indeed, the evidence points to the fact that most of these techniques bring with them the great risk of suggestion.

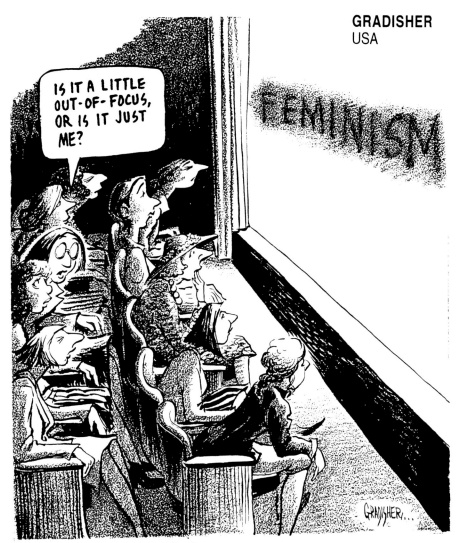

Gradisher/Cartoonists & Writers Syndicate

The feminist movement holds wide appeal for most women. Many of the mothers who have been accused of being perpetrators or enablers by their daughters in this recovered memory phenomenon are feminists. So are their daughters. But their views of feminism are widely separated. The mothers view feminism as a method of thinking that liberated women and expanded their possibilities.

Feminism provided support for them to become doctors, teachers, writers, mothers and wives at the same time. Many of these women are grateful to Betty Friedan and Gloria Steinem, leaders in the women's movement, who spread the notion that women could and should do all things. Consciousness raising groups helped these women lessen their isolation and strengthen their commitment to political altruism through mutual revelations of common experiences. These groups, which originated as a structured series of meetings by and for women, brought new recruits to feminist ideology. For many women, the group experience opened their minds to all sorts of possibilities.

The women's movement was always home for a wide range of ideas. While many women with husbands and children join feminist groups, so do women who choose the single life.

Part of the women's movement is called gender feminism. In its extreme, it is a movement that claims Western civilization is a patriarchal society in which men rule women by force, using rape as a weapon. There are many books that expound upon this point of view.

Sonia Johnson is a leader of what might be called gender feminism.

Johnson joined the women's movement in the 1970s when the Mormon Church, to which she belonged, opposed the Equal Rights Amendment. She formed Mormons for the ERA and later ran for U.S. president. Her book Going Out of Our Minds *addresses feminist spirituality. She recommends group meditation or "self-hypnosis" to gain understanding of the pervasive nature of male domination or patriarchy. She sees herself and all like-minded women as prophets and believes that only by "going out of our minds" can women*

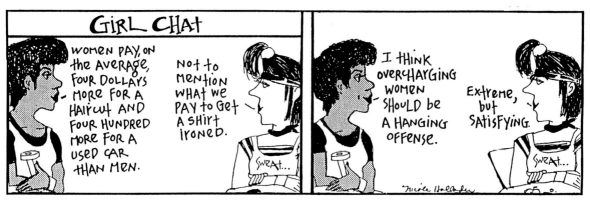

GIRL CHAT

WOMEN PAY, ON the AVERAGE, FOUR DOLLARS MORE FOR A HAIRCUT AND FOUR HUNDRED MORE FOR A USED CAR THAN MEN.

Not to mention WHAT WE PAY to Get A SHIRT IRONED.

SWEAT...

I THINK OVERCHARGING WOMEN SHOULD be A HANGING OFFENSE.

Extreme, but SATISFYING.

SWEAT...

Hollander/Cartoonists & Writers Syndicate

HOLLANDER USA

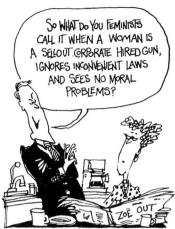
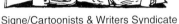
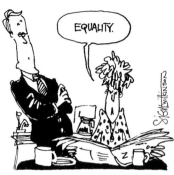

Signe/Cartoonists & Writers Syndicate

SIGNE USA

patriarchy's scorn—the immense and various resources of my spirit and deep mind.

Hand in hand now let us leap off this stinking rubbish heap men call "civilization," out of our limited, lightless, dying patriarchal minds, and reach for our lives— for all life—deep into the cosmos that is our own souls.[2]

Another book with influence in the gender feminist movement is the *Great Cosmic Mother* by Monica Sjöö and Barbara Mor.

This book is credited with showing that the religion of the Goddess is our ancient heritage. The religion of the Goddess "is tied to the cycles of women's bodies, the seasons, the phases of the moon, and the fertility of the earth—was the original religion of all humanity." Sjöö is an artist and theoretician of the Goddess religion. Mor is an American poet.[3]

The following passages from their book speak for themselves:

Reich pointed out in the 1930s that the prevalent male sexual fantasy in male-dominated society, is one of rape.

And it confirms what too many people do not want to know: that the first "God" was female.

Truly, our very sanity is at stake with continuing patriarchy and the denial of the cosmic self—the Goddess—within us all, and us within her.

Women who cannot or will not accept taboos are still punished, as we've been punished for two thousand years in the

boycott patriarchy *"emotionally, spiritually, and intellectually" and thus transform society. Not only does patriarchy rule the world, it destroys the soul of women because it allows men full control over them.*[1]

The following are quotes from *Going Out of Our Minds*:

We have not been warned that Daddy is our enemy, or Grandpa, or Uncle Steve, or brother Harvey.

Like rape, despite rhetoric to the contrary, incest is not only encouraged, it is insisted upon; not just condoned, but blessed.

Like rape, incest is not accidental. It is an institution *of patriarchy—like the church, like the law: absolutely necessary to maintaining male privilege and power.*

Not with fear and dread, but with hope and love, we can leap out of our minds, free of patriarchy, into a celebration of life. I believe there is no other way.

I decided that this time out I am going to begin to learn to use—despite

85

patriarchal world–as Lesbians, unmarried mothers, thinkers, artists, witches. One form of punishment is culturally mandated rape.

Women, in the Judeo-Christian-Islamic-Buddhist-Hindu-Confucian traditions, are seen as some kind of functional mistake. Nature is a mistake. Life is a mistake. And the male mind was born to correct it.[4]

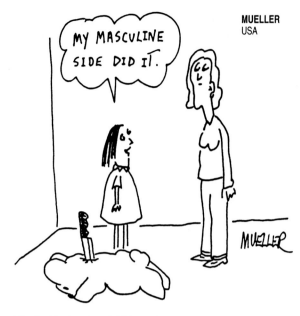

MUELLER
USA

Mueller/Cartoonists & Writers Syndicate

Gloria Finds Self-Esteem

Many women who are mothers of these adult children feel gratitude for Gloria Steinem's courage to speak out and champion their causes. "She was a role-model: articulate, intelligent, energetic, ambitious, and attractive. She seemed to have reached the pinnacle of success–one of the best-known, revered women in the world."[5] But as discussed earlier, Steinem was not a happy person. Most of those years while carrying the banner for women, she was riddled with self-doubt and anguish, lacking self-esteem. However, she bared her soul in her book *Revolution from Within.* She has discovered her "inner child." This inner child had been destroyed by the patriarchal society in which we live. Steinem has embraced the tenets of Recovery, New Age and gender feminism. The women who gave her their honor and respect in the 1970s and 1980s will find a new Steinem in the 1990s–one who is less pragmatic and more spiritual. She provides a complete rationale for gender feminism using the constructs of Recovery and New Age.

Steinem discusses "voyaging to time past,"[6] quoting John Bradshaw: "I believe that this neglected, wounded inner child of the past is the major source of human misery."[7]

In order to find her inner child and reparent herself, Steinem visits a psychotherapist whom she says is "an experienced travel guide for journeys into the unconscious–that timeless part of our minds where events and emotions of our personal past are stored along with the wisdom of our species."[8]

The feminist movement changed American society, it empowered women and created a revolution. But like all revolutions, it had a down side. In the gender feminist movement, men are perceived as opponents. So it is not a surprise that many innocent men have been swept up in a witch hunt, accused of atrocious crimes they did not commit in the wave of hysteria that accompanied this revolution.

CHAPTER 21—SATANIC RITUAL ABUSE

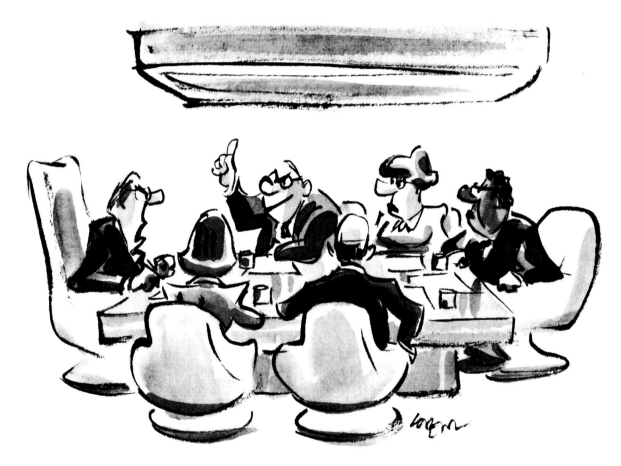

"*Now, just a darn minute, Fowler! You're not the only member of this board who was a victim of ritual satanic abuse!*"

Drawing by Lorenz; © 1993 The New Yorker Magazine, Inc.

In a 1990 broadcast segment on "Ritual Abuse," psychologist Sophia Carr, Ph.D., told an Oregon audience that she had been physically and sexually tortured at age 13 near her home in Bremerton, Washington. She described six men wearing medallions, dressed in robes, who took her to an altar and recited chants. But before they could cut out her heart, the horse she had been riding came back and scared the men away.

In 1992, one of Carr's patients, Jennifer Fultz, "remembered" that she was lying on a concrete slab surrounded by men in animal skins. She recalled her mother watching as the men raped her. Later, the men aborted her fetus and told her, "Eat its flesh." In 1994, Jennifer filed a lawsuit against Carr and her associate Chyril Walker. In 1996, Walker settled for more than $1.15 million and Carr settled for an undisclosed amount.[1]

This sequence of events illustrates the cycle of the satanic scare that swept the country during the 1980s. As Eleanor Goldstein and Kevin Farmer noted in their book *Confabulations*:

> At about the same time that therapy-induced memories of childhood incest became common, grotesque stories of ritualistic abuse by satanic cults began emerging from therapy sessions. A growing number of licensed therapists are involved in these cases. Some therapists claim that they have patients who are victims of an international cult of satanists operating in virtually every town and city in America. Satanists, they claimed, have infiltrated the highest ranks of government, law enforce-

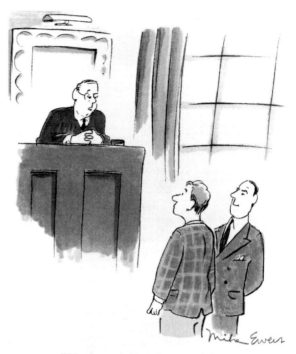

"Ritual satanic abuse is a powerful defense, Mr. Lewis. Are you sure you want to blow it on parking violations?"

ment and other professions useful to guarding the secret conspiracy.[2]

Co-author of *The Courage to Heal*, Laura Davis, in a book, *Allies in Healing*, tells her readers:

> Cult abuse has far-reaching effects on its victims. In addition to the problems most survivors of sexual abuse and incest already experience, cult abuse survivors also have to deal with the results of brainwashing, severe intimidation, extreme humiliation, sensory deprivation, starvation, forced drug experiences, extreme torture, and the trauma of witnessing or being forced to participate in ritual murders or abuse of animals or other children.[3]

Satanic ritual abuse (SRA) beliefs were not restricted to pop-psychology or "fringe" therapists. Mary Shanley spent three years in psychiatric wards diagnosed as a victim of satanic ritual abuse. She said, "[My doctors] told me that I had already been programmed that if I divulged the secrets from the cult that I would self-destruct and that my programming had just been turned on at age 39. . . . They were the experts."[4] Mary has since sued the doctors who diagnosed her as a survivor of SRA, and she received a large settlement in 1996.

Pat Burgus turned to the prestigious Rush Presbyterian Hospital in Chicago and to Dr. Bennett Braun when she needed help. She came to believe that she was the Satanic High Priestess of a nine-state region. Pat was kept in a psychiatric ward for 1,200 days. Claiming it was for their own protection, Braun hospitalized Burgus' 5-year-old and 4-year-old sons in a children's psychiatric unit at Rush for approximately three years. Braun has said that "satanic ritual abusers are part of an 'international organization that's got a structure somewhat similar to that of the Communist cell.'"[5] Burgus filed a lawsuit against Braun which was settled out of court for $10.6 million in favor of Burgus.[6]

Satanic rumors have cropped up periodically since the Middle Ages.[7] The current wave of satanic belief started in 1980 with the publication of *Michelle Remembers* by Michelle Smith and Dr. Lawrence Pazder. Set in British Columbia, this may be the oldest known Satanic cult "survivor" testimonial.

In 1983, rumors that Satanists were sexually molesting children in day care centers began to appear in the McMartin Preschool case in Manhattan Beach, California.[8] Dr. Pazder had explained his theories

OUTLAND   **BY BERKELY BREATHED**

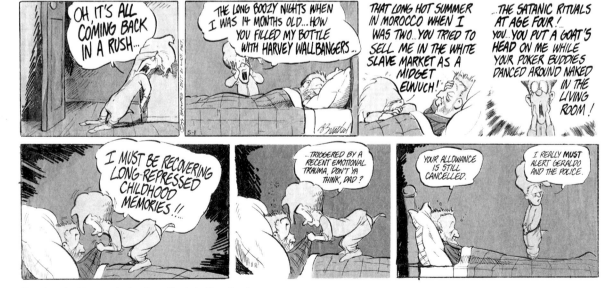

Reprinted with permission from Berkely Breathed.

to the parents and therapists in that case.[9]

A national network of investigators, therapists, social workers, doctors, preachers, prosecutors and others helped to create the recent hysteria that devil worshippers are killing babies, impregnating little girls and forcing bizarre and violent acts of sexual and physical abuse on children. Newspapers reported every exaggerated incident as if it were real. Geraldo Rivera, Sally Jessy Rafael and other popular television personalities had millions of people believing these confabulated tales by giving proponents of this satanic conspiracy a national forum. Since the early 1980s, hundreds of cases have been investigated. Many people have been charged with crimes and imprisoned.

Eventually, people realized that there was no evidence for the horrific crimes being described. According to FBI agent and chief investigator of crimes against children, Kenneth V. Lanning:

We live in a very violent society, and yet we have "only" about 23,000 murders a year. Those who accept these stories of mass human sacrifice would have us believe that the satanists and other occult practitioners are murdering more than twice as many people every year.[10]

SRA started to get bad press and in 1991, the term "sadistic abuse" was introduced.

In 1994, the first empirical study of the prevalence of SRA was published. Based on information from district attorneys, social service workers, police officials and psychotherapists, the study suggests that these tales are usually figments of imagination.[11]

This federally commissioned research project, directed by Gail Goodman, Ph.D., examined 12,264 cases of suspected SRA.

The research could not find a single case of alleged child sexual abuse where there was clear corroborating evidence for the existence of a well-organized inter-generational satanic cult which tortured children and committed murders.[12]

Unfortunately, the belief in SRA has caused much harm and cost much money. In the spring of 1996, a study of some Victim's Compensation Program claimants in Washington state was released. Of 30 cases that were randomly selected for closer examination, 29 reported memories of satanic ritual abuse. The number of murders reported by this group was 150, yet no corroboration was ever sought. No medical evidence was ever found to corroborate their claims of torture or mutilation.[13]

Before they recovered memories, only three claimants thought about suicide. After they recovered memories, 20 contemplated killing themselves. In fact, the results were so disturbing that the state of Washington has amended its Victim Compensation program and no longer funds the kind of therapy that produced the SRA memories.[14]

Skepticism is growing about the claims of intergenerational satanic abuse. While it is still possible to find workshops about treating SRA victims, and while there are still books being published, there are fewer each year. We seem to be on the downside of a satanic panic very similar to those that have periodically swept through societies since the Middle Ages.

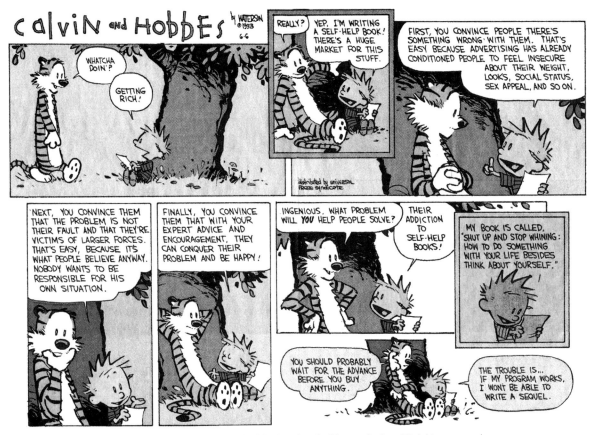

The recovery movement is big business. With 10 to 25 million admitted alcoholics in the 1980s, a huge marketplace was identified.

Being a member of a 12-Step Support Group became a status symbol. According to Carla Wills-Brandon, an author of six recovery books:

During the middle [80s] the media was all [abuzz] with the Recovery Movement and recovery jargon. The producers of television talk shows would call publicity agencies looking for the gurus and authors of self help books to appear on their shows. The media quickly realized that airing dysfunctional laundry on national radio or television was good for business.[1]

Wills-Brandon was on the "inside of the movement looking out."[2] She says:

Television wasn't the only member of the media looking to make a quick buck off the Recovery Movement. Numerous newspapers were clamoring for stories about recovery from everything from manic depression, alcoholism, and bulimia to physical abuse and sexual moles-

tation. The more sensational, the better. This made great copy and sold tons of newspapers, especially if the story was about a celebrity in recovery.[3]

Fueling the sale of books and other paraphernalia for 12-Steppers was a proliferation of seminars around the world. "In 1990, Health Communications, Inc. (HCI) was sponsoring about 17 or 18 regional conferences and one national conference every year; it was also venturing out internationally, with conferences in Canada and Australia."[4]

Health Communications, Inc. is a publishing company in Deerfield Beach, Florida, founded by Gary Seidler and Peter Vegso who moved to Florida from Canada in the late 1970s to found *The U.S. Journal of Addictions.* They soon branched out from the *Journal* to magazines, to book publishing, to seminars. HCI published the first book on codependency in 1983, which rapidly became a *New York Times* best seller, entitled *Adult Children of Alcoholics.* The author, Janet Geringer Woititz, is considered the mother of codependency.

Hi and Lois

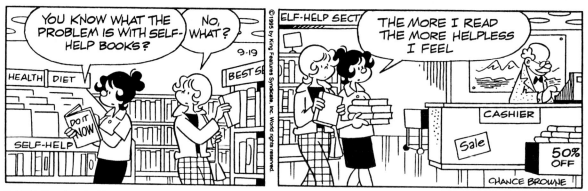

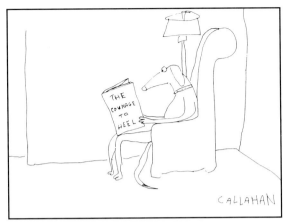

Reprinted courtesy of Levin Represents.

This book is reputed to have sold at least 2 million copies.

HCI was also the publisher for John Bradshaw's first book, published in 1988, entitled *Bradshaw On: The Family.* Bradshaw, a former minister, had several series on PBS, which was a tremendous way to encourage book sales. Before long, HCI had about 200 paperback titles, and the gurus who wrote their books were on the road regularly promoting their books and holding conference seminars. HCI also published *Changes Magazine,* which was an advertising vehicle for seminars and rehab centers, many of which were supported by insurance at rates of $1,000 a day.

Bradshaw's popularity led him to bigger publishers with bigger advances.

Along with the large expenditures now being paid for books, treatment centers and seminars (many offering continuing education credits), there was the growth of the support industry, providing coffee cups (coffee is big with AA members), greeting cards, cuddly toys, T-shirts and blankets.

After all, every thoughtful adult child needs to comfort his inner child with at least a teddy bear.

The power of books cannot be overestimated. *The Courage to Heal* by Ellen Bass and Laura Davis, has sold well over a million copies. The book, and its accompanying workbook by Laura Davis, has influenced countless people. Its theory is that if your life shows the symptoms (and there are many) you have been abused, even if you don't remember. Parents find that prescriptions for cutting off from families, as described in the books, have been carried out in real life and they are victims of the advice given in this most notorious of all self-help books, which has been a source of great income to the authors and their publishers.

In 1992 Wendy Kaminer wrote:

Imagine America without self-help books. Imagine everyone grappling with their problems and forging their identities, using their own intuitions and powers of analysis and maybe some help from their friends. Imagine that. I can't. I have no cure for America's self-help habit and no advice to offer on how to find one. . . . I have no expectations that the "problem" of self-help ever will be solved. Instead, I expect more self-help books, not less, now that publishers have a broad new market to exploit— wanna-be-"wild" middle-class men.

Codependency books may soon be as passé as last year's diet, but the self-help genre will always be in fashion. Self-help books market authority in a culture that idealizes individualism but

93

NON SEQUITUR

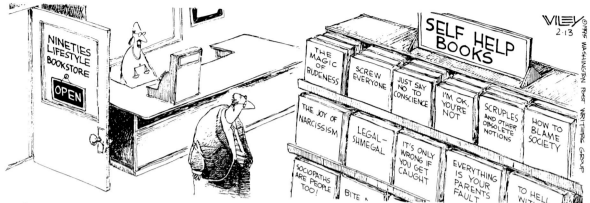

not thinking, and fears the isolation of being free. "A book must be the axe for the frozen sea within us," Kafka wrote.

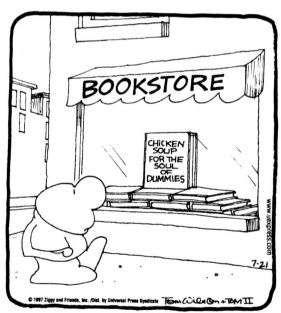

Self-help is how we skate.[5]

In 1994, I* visited Seidler and Vegso at their facility in Deerfield Beach, Florida.[6] The company had hit on hard times. Their recovery book sales had suffered a steep decline. Gary Seidler said to me, "Recovery is dead. We are looking for a new best seller." They found it! Unless you've been on another planet, you've seen HCI's new best seller *Chicken Soup for the Soul,* which is a publishing phenomenon. There are about half-a-dozen books in the series, from a *Second Helping of Chicken Soup,* up to about the fourth serving. Then there's *Chicken Soup for Teens, Condensed Chicken Soup* and a *Chicken Soup Cookbook.*

A new trend seems to be emerging from which much money is being made—one that offers feel-good sentiments. Let's hope it can overcome some of the damage that is the fallout of the obsessive aspects of the recovery movement.

* Eleanor Goldstein is the author of this chapter.

94

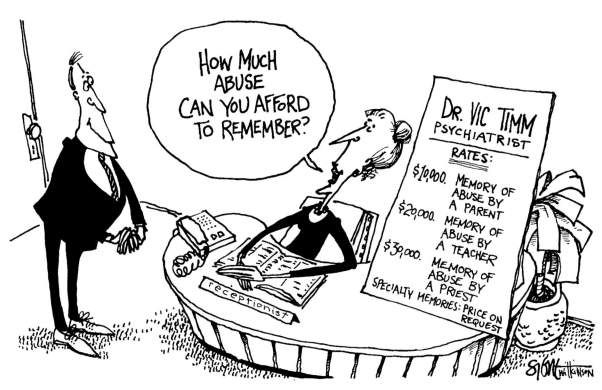

SIGNE
PHILADELPHIA DAILY NEWS
Philadelphia
USA

SIGNE/Cartoonists & Writers Syndicate

Until the mid-1970s, most therapists were either on a salary from an institution with which they were affiliated or they received a fee for their services. Then the laws changed and health insurance coverage was broadened to include mental health treatment. Referred to as "third-party" payments, insurance payments for mental health coverage exploded through the 1980s. So did the number of people who decided to become therapists.

Professional schools of psychology started to churn out practitioners and many social workers began to provide individual psychotherapy. The field of Marriage and Family Counseling (MFC) was established and by 1989, California alone had 23,000 people certified in this field.[1]

States expanded the number of professionals who were "licensed" and thus eligible to receive third-party payment from insurance companies. School counseling, pastoral counseling, and drug and alcohol counseling all attracted practitioners. Suddenly there were more therapists than the market could absorb.

According to Tana Dineen: "Now psychologists of different persuasions vie for the limited health dollars and openly and aggressively compete amongst themselves for clients."[2]

In 1985, the federal government removed restrictions on the building of new mental health facilities. During the 1980s, profits in U.S. private psychiatric hospitals surged from less than $1 billion to nearly $7 billion.[3]

The psychiatric industry used aggressive marketing to fill hospital beds with patients covered by expanded mental health insurance employee benefits. Some of the marketing was direct and some indirect. Hot lines for this or that disorder, free evaluations, special programs for gamblers, professional women, the overweight or the underweight, the depressed, persons who "might" be abused—all drew people to hospitals. Some hospitals even paid bounties to recruiters in schools, businesses or counseling centers that sent patients to them.

Some believed they were going to a vacation resort. One patient originally sought treatment for a neck injury. An-

Up and Running

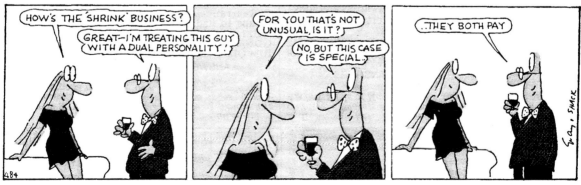

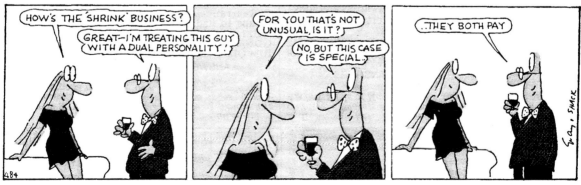© 1997. Reprinted with permission from Solo Syndications.

other wanted help for a weight problem.

Instead, they all were committed to Florida psychiatric hospitals, victims of a national insurance fraud scam ... that paid kickbacks to employee assistance plan administrators and others to lure patients to their facilities.[4]

"Psychiatric Hospitals Accused of Fraud"
***Miami Herald,* December 21, 1996**

Overweight and suffering from stress, the New Yorker [Michael Jones] had flown cross-country to attend what was advertised as a weight-loss clinic in sunny Southern California. The air fare was free and the treatment, he was told, fully covered by his Blue Cross plan.

But when Michael reached Los Angeles, he was shocked to find himself booked into a psychiatric hospital.

Michael's is one of many stories emerging from federal and state lawsuits in Los Angeles in which insurers accuse A Place for Us *of enlisting doctors and hospital staff to falsify diagnoses and medical records in order to obtain payment for treatment.[5]*

"Diet Clinic Tactics Draw Fire"
***Los Angeles Times,* April 10, 1994**

Between 1987 and 1993, the cost per employee of the average company's mental-health bill actually doubled.[6] The field developed so quickly that insurance companies began to try to contain the unrestrained growth in mental health payments. Some instituted computer programs to track the effectiveness of particular treatments for certain diagnoses. Some corporations moved to managed-care networks and health maintenance organizations (HMOs) began to take

QUALITY TIME   Gail Machlis

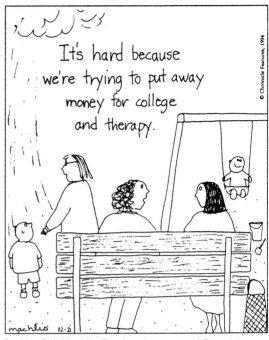

It's hard because we're trying to put away money for college and therapy.

on a large part of the health market in an effort to restrain all health costs.

The increase in costs was so dramatic that Texas Attorney General Dan Morales initiated the first of many state investigations around the country. The investigations in Texas showed widespread patterns of abuse—all aimed at milking insurance policies—among the nation's therapists and mental-health hospitals. This was followed by an investigation, which included the FBI and other federal agencies, into the workings of private psychiatric hospitals across the country.[7]

In 1993, the first large chain to be sued was the National Medical Enterprises (NME) organization. Offices in hospitals were raided by the FBI and other federal agents who had been investigating them for

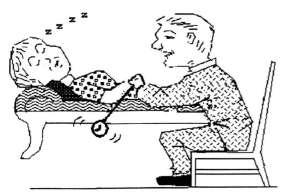

Now you are going into the future. It's the end of the month. Have you paid your account?

several years and evidence was found that NME had undertaken a coordinated national scheme to hospitalize thousands of patients who did not need to be hospitalized.[8] Newspaper stories and television documentaries highlight the huge amounts of money that were paid to private hospitals for patients who were "recovering memories."

In a suit filed late Friday, Shanley accuses Houston psychologist Judith Peterson and doctors and hospitals in Texas and Indiana of conspiracy, negligence and fraud in connection with her 3½ years of therapy that cost her insurance company more than $2 million.[9]

"Suit Hits Satanism Memories"
Houston Chronicle, December 13, 1994

Lynn Carl, now of Baltimore, said she spent more than $2 million on mental health treatment after therapists at Spring Shadows Glen Psychiatric Hospital convinced her she was a Satan worshiper ritually abused since childhood.[10]

"Woman Sues Therapists Over 500 Personalities Claim"
Houston Chronicle, March 8, 1995

Pat Burgus: Our 5-year-old, John, who went in, was there for 39 months and Mikey was brought into the hospital 4 years old and he was kept on a children's psychiatric unit for 32 months. From the time I entered the hospital until we got the children out of the hospital by court order, it was 1,200 days.

Interviewer: And how much money?

Pat Burgus: We each had $1 million insurance policy that was almost completely topped out. So we're looking at $3 million.[11]

"Search for Satan"
Frontline Documentary, October 1995

As insurance companies started to get a grip on the exploding costs, they set limits on reimbursements and they stated that some therapies are needlessly time consuming and empirically untested. In some states, managed-care networks have reduced the average private therapist's income by nearly 50%. This will likely spur research in testing the effectiveness of various therapies so that we know what works, with whom and under what conditions.

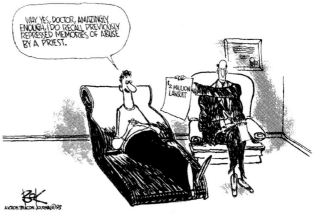

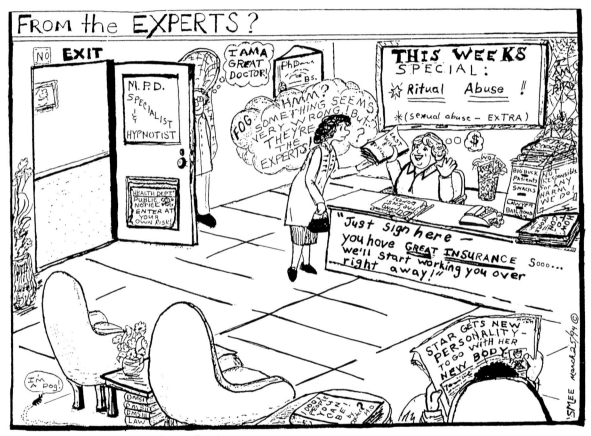

Reprinted with permission from Sharon Gornic.

Insurance drives every aspect of the "False Memory Syndrome" (FMS) phenomenon. Private health insurance pays for therapy. Social security and victims' compensation—insurance of the last resort—pay for therapy when private insurance monies are depleted. Parents have been sued through their homeowner's insurance to pay for therapy. Malpractice insurance pays claims to former patients.

Private insurance coverage for mental health is a recent trend. It took hold in the 1980s when many generous plans agreed to pay for alcohol recovery programs. Treatment centers sprouted up across the land. Even some popular 1970s Arizona dude ranches were reborn as alcohol recovery centers.

Then, at the end of the 1980s, because of out-of-control escalating costs, insurance companies discontinued their generous payments for recovery programs. A new market was needed to maintain facilities and income levels. Recovery patients were replaced by survivors and multiple personality patients who had been diagnosed with Post-traumatic Stress Disorder or Dissociative Identity Disorder. These diagnoses continued to be covered by insurance because they were listed in the *Diagnostic and Statistical Manual (DSM III)*.

Treatment for survivors and for MPD patients takes a long time and often the patients don't seem to get any better. August Piper has noted:

This apparent lack of progress persists in spite of the expenditure of huge sums on their treatment, the amassing of untold hours of psychotherapy, and the utilization of numerous hospital stays that are sufficient to generate charts a foot or more thick in just a few years.[1]

The American Psychiatric Association noted, "Favorable prognosis of MPD requires intensive treatment . . . over a protracted period of time."[2] In fact, the treatment of Sybil, whose story was discussed in Chapter 17, required 11 years of therapy and more than 2,300 office visits.[3]

When insurance coverage for survivors is exhausted, patients need to find means to pay for their therapy. *The Courage to Heal* informs "survivors" that if they file a lawsuit against their parents, they can expect

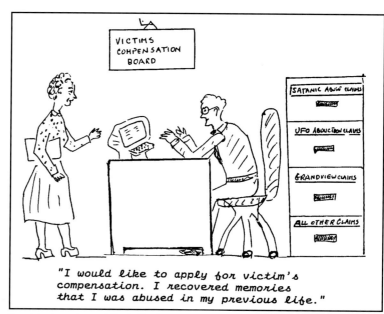

"I would like to apply for victim's compensation. I recovered memories that I was abused in my previous life."

Reprinted courtesy of Paula Tyroler.

BALLARD STREET

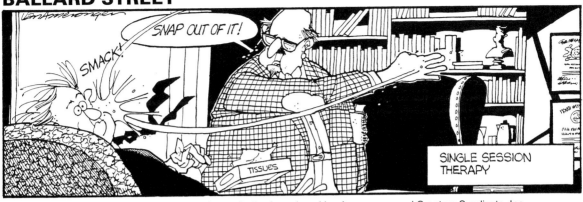

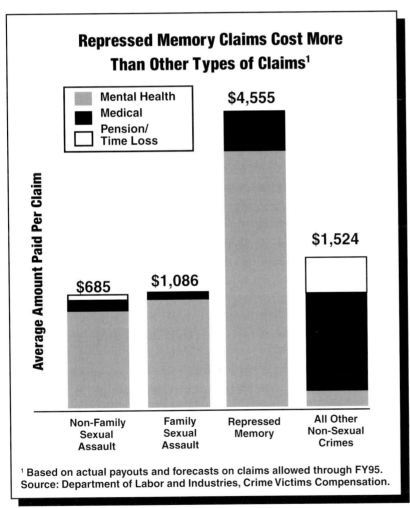

Repressed Memory Claims Cost More Than Other Types of Claims[1]

Legend:
- Mental Health (gray)
- Medical (black)
- Pension/Time Loss (white)

Average Amount Paid Per Claim

Non-Family Sexual Assault	Family Sexual Assault	Repressed Memory	All Other Non-Sexual Crimes
$685	$1,086	$4,555	$1,524

[1] Based on actual payouts and forecasts on claims allowed through FY95.
Source: Department of Labor and Industries, Crime Victims Compensation.

These statistics are from the state of Washington and are a microcosm of the United States at large.

payment through their parents' homeowner insurance policy. *The Courage to Heal* even includes a list of lawyers who will file such suits.[4]

Social security disability and victims' compensation are other ways to pay for therapy when private insurance monies have expired. The records of some retractors indicate that their therapists had certified them as disabled. Thus, they qualified for disability payments and their therapy was paid for by Social Security.

Another route to government insurance money for therapy has been through the victims' compensation programs that are administered by individual states. Victims' compensation

FARCUS

by David Waisglass
& Gordon Coulhart

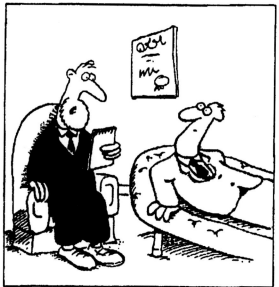

"Do all your multiple personalities have health plans?"

programs are for victims of crimes, and child abuse is a crime. Washington state was the first state to change its statute of limitations on claims for past sexual abuse and to cover "survivors." That state has provided the most comprehensive information on the extremely expensive costs of recovered memory therapy.[5]

In 1994, the Ramona case hit the news wires. Gary Ramona's daughter, Holly, sued him for sexual abuse. He later sued Holly's therapist and the hospital where she was told that "memories" elicited during a sodium amytal interview were historically accurate. Ramona won his case, receiving $500,000.[6] This was the first third-party case against a therapist due to false memories, and it sent shock waves through the malpractice insur-

ance industry.[7]

One insurance firm tripled the cost of malpractice insurance for therapists.[8] According to California attorney Brandt Caudill, "legal experts estimate that as many as 17,000 claims against mental health professionals may be filed in the next ten years at a cost of over $250 million in litigation costs."[9]

In 1996, one major insurer announced that it will no longer provide malpractice coverage for anyone who uses "hypno-therapy to assist clients in recovering failed or repressed memories of possible abuse."[10]

In the past year, headlines have highlighted another part of the insurance story.

$1 Million Awarded to Settle Lawsuit—A State Farm Payout Ends the Suit Against a Local Assembly of God[11]
—Rutherford lawsuit, November 1996

2nd Patient Wins Against Psychiatrist: Accusation of Planting Memories Brings Multimillion Dollar Verdict[12]
—Humenansky case, January 1996

Jury Awards $5.8 Million in Satanic Memories Case[13]
—Carl lawsuit, August 1997

Woman Wins $10 M in False Memory Suit[14]
—Burgus lawsuit, November 1997

Former patients are suing recovered memory therapists and receiving large malpractice awards. This will contribute to recovered memory therapy's eventual demise.

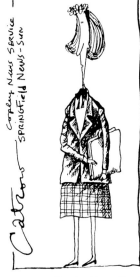

MY THERAPIST helped me recover long repressed memories of years of child abuse at the hands of my parents —

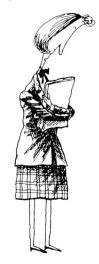

I'm certain they screamed and beat me and humiliated me in horrible and unspeakable ways —How else can I explain the way I turned out...

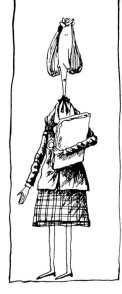

So we went to the police and had them charged

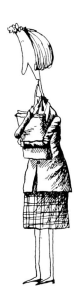

My therapist says I'm just in denial and my doubts will pass...

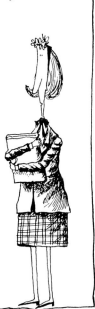

...just as soon as the GUILTY are Behind bars

I magine receiving the following letter "out of the blue:"

Dear Mr. and Mrs. "R",

Please be advised that this Law Firm represents your daughter. She has consulted with me regarding the effects she is suffering from severe childhood trauma resulting from the abuse inflicted by you. The trauma described is unspeakable. As a result of this trauma, without relating all of the details in this letter, she has been unable to hold a full-time job. . . . Without filing a Court action, Ms. "R" has authorized me to make the following demand letter for settlement:

1. *You assume responsibility for Ms. "R's" medical and therapeutic expenses including any hospitalization for the remainder of her life.*
2. *Reimbursement to Ms."R" for therapy and hospitalization expenses incurred during 1990 and 1991, in the estimated amount of $10,000.*
3. *Payment of $250,000 to help, in some small way, to compensate her for the disabilities, pain, suffering, humiliation and severe lifetime trauma that she has suffered and is expected to suffer.*
4. *A life insurance policy to be taken out on your lives with Ms. "R" to be named as beneficiary to ensure that the settlement be paid.*

If I do not hear from you within 10 days, I will assume that you do not intend to enter into settlement and will advise Ms. "R" regarding the appropriate judicial relief. Rest assured, however, that if you do not settle this matter, in any lawsuit, Ms. "R" will be requesting substantially higher sums and her attorney's fees. As a lawyer, I have dealt with many of these cases, and the facts that have been related to me and which will be related to a jury, warrant the imposition of substantial punitive and compensatory damages.

Your daughter's lawyer[1]

Hundreds of families have received similar demand letters. Some families paid because they were fearful for their jobs or reputations. Some of the families ignored the letters and nothing happened. Other families were sued.

One of the first repressed memory civil lawsuits was brought to trial in California in 1991. A 74-year-old widowed grandmother and retired registered nurse was accused of satanically ritually abusing her two daughters, ages 48 and 35, and a grandchild. A masters level counselor who never looked at their medical records made the diagnosis for all three "victims" within one month after the eldest daughter told him that she thought she had Multiple Personality Disorder on May 15, 1988. The

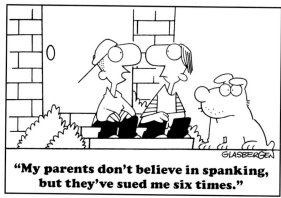

"My parents don't believe in spanking, but they've sued me six times."

© 1996 Randy Glasbergen. Reprinted with permission.

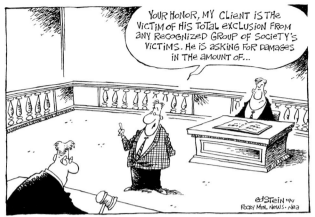

YOUR HONOR, MY CLIENT IS THE VICTIM OF HIS TOTAL EXCLUSION FROM ANY RECOGNIZED GROUP OF SOCIETY'S VICTIMS. HE IS ASKING FOR DAMAGES IN THE AMOUNT OF...

edSTEIN '94
Rocky Mtn. News·Nea

counselor had no training in Multiple Personality Disorder, but he had read some books including *Michelle Remembers*. The case went to jury. No money was awarded to the plaintiffs.[2]

The idea of suing an abuser seems to have spread from the book, *The Courage to Heal*: "There are nonviolent means of retribution you can seek."[3] It is the ultimate confrontation. "Suing your abuser and turning him in to the authorities are just two of the avenues open."[4]

It became a possibility for "adult survivors" to sue when states began to change their statutes of limitations to allow for "repressed memories." The first repressed memory criminal case was the much publicized trial of George Franklin in 1991. Franklin was accused of a murder that had occurred 20 years earlier based only on evidence of his daughter's recovered memory. Franklin was convicted and spent five years in jail until his conviction was overturned. In 1996, prosecutors decided not to retry Franklin when it was learned

that his daughter had retrieved her memories with the aid of hypnosis, and that he could not possibly have committed a second murder for which she also accused him.[5]

In June 1997, George Franklin filed a lawsuit against his daughter. The prosecutors and expert witness Dr. Lenore Terr admitted to conspiring to convict him.[6]

By 1992, the National Organization of Women made available a *Legal Resource Kit on Incest and Child Sexual Abuse*. The paper notes that many adult victims have no idea of what happened to them as children until they recall the details "through the help of therapy or life events."[7]

It goes on to say:

Civil legal remedies are crucial to deter these acts, to punish wrongdoers, and to try to compensate the victim for her injuries, including providing her with funds for much-needed medical and psychological treatment. Most important, allowing incest survivors their "day in court" will empower them and prove to society at large that violent male tyranny over female family members will not be tolerated.[8]

In 1992, lawyers Joseph and Kimberly Crnich wrote a whole book on how to sue in these cases.

A creative lawyer can sometimes make other claims against your perpetrator, such as deceit or defamation, to recover against the insurance company. In some cases, suing a parent who was not the direct abuser but did not stop it (often the mother) is another possible way to receive insurance coverage.[9]

The notion of "lawsuits as therapy" was short-lived. Indeed, lawsuits of another nature began to be filed, starting around 1994. These were civil lawsuits brought against therapists by former patients who claimed that they had acquired false memories in therapy. They claimed they had not been informed that memories which develop with the use of hypnosis may be unreliable. They charged they had been subjected to experimental techniques for which they had not given informed consent.

In the fall of 1997, five psychiatric workers were *criminally* indicted by a Houston federal grand jury for collecting millions of dollars in fraudulent insurance payments. Two psychiatrists, a psychologist, a therapist, and a hospital administrator were accused of using "brainwashing" techniques on psychiatric patients to help them "recover" bizarre memories of cannibalism, torture and human sacrifice. These memories were then frequently used to document false diagnoses of multiple personality disorder in patients with large insurance policies.[10]

The law has been involved in diverse aspects of the recovered/repressed memory controversy.

In 1993, the FMS Foundation began to track the legal cases that were brought to its attention. In an examination of more

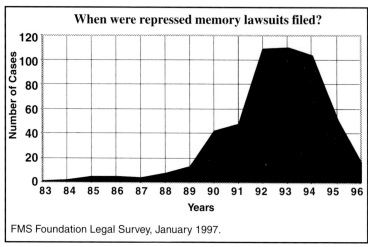

When were repressed memory lawsuits filed?

FMS Foundation Legal Survey, January 1997.

than 500 cases in which the *only* evidence was a recovered repressed memory, it appears that 15% of the repressed memory cases filed were criminal suits and 85% were civil suits. There was a precipitous rise in such cases between 1989 and 1992, and an equally sharp drop starting in 1994.[11] In 1992, it was likely that these cases would go to court or be settled out of court. This has changed. It is now more likely for a repressed memory claim to be dropped, dismissed or withdrawn than to go to trial.

A number of descriptions or case histories have been published about the experiences of people who have sued. They show that the standards of fact in the legal system are far different than the standards in therapy. As a consequence, it appears that most of the adult children who brought these suits ended up with nothing and were abandoned by their families.

The notion of "lawsuits as therapy" was short-lived.

The Panic Is Subsiding

"We have come a long way from tears to laughter." —A Dad

In March 1992, a handful of families and professionals came together and formed the False Memory Syndrome (FMS) Foundation. Parents wanted to try to understand why their now adult children had shown such a dramatic change of behavior. The families also wanted to help each other cope with being falsely accused of incest and with the awful pain of the loss of their children. They came together just as parents of Down's syndrome children or parents of children with sickle cell anemia or parents of children who had joined cults have come together for mutual support.

By 1997, about 18,000 affected families contacted the FMS Foundation from every state, including Alaska and Hawaii, and from Guam and Puerto Rico. Families have also made contact from Australia, Brazil, Canada, Chile, Denmark, England, Germany, Israel, Japan, Mexico, Netherlands, Norway, Philippines, Sweden, South Africa and New Zealand.

The FMS Foundation has served as a clearinghouse for information about the recovered/repressed memory debate. It has

FEIFFER®

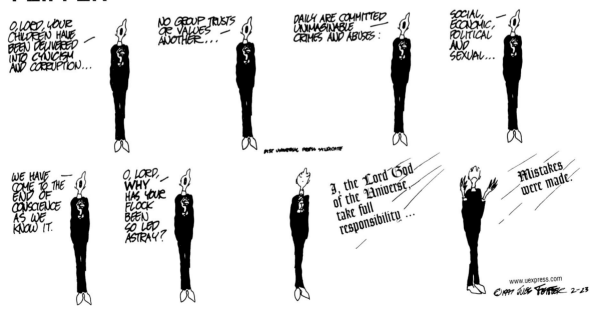

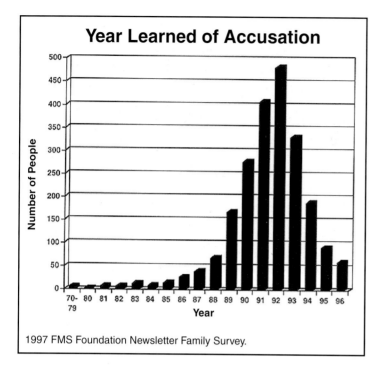

Year Learned of Accusation

1997 FMS Foundation Newsletter Family Survey.

threat is either non-existent or greatly exaggerated. . . . A moral panic is long-lasting and gives rise to organizations, laws, and procedures to combat the perceived threat.[1]

A number of professionals have come to view the recovered memory movement within this context.

In January 1997, over 2,000 families (61%) who were members of the FMS Foundation responded to a short survey. Their answers provide a sharp picture of the FMS situation.[2]

Gender of Accuser:
Male: 8.43%   Female: 91.57%

Was the accuser in therapy when accusations were made?
Yes: 91.82%   No: 2.71%
Don't know: 5.47%

Did the accusations involve "repressed" memories?
Yes: 92.62%   No: 1.41%
Don't know: 5.98%

Families also reported on the year in which they learned about the accusation. The chart below shows a sudden rise and fall that looks like some change in practice or in culture—or both—has taken place. The alleged events of abuse were supposed to have occurred over many years, several decades ago. We would expect the reporting to cover a similar time span.

One possible interpretation of this data is

documented the passage of the phenomenon by archiving professional publications, newspaper and magazine articles, advertisements, cartoons and videotape programs. The Foundation also conducted several surveys to learn about the families who had been accused.

What was learned about these families supports an understanding of the recovered memory movement as a social phenomenon. Sociologists have studied other mass delusions or moral panics and learned about the conditions that support them and how they spread. As sociologist Jeffrey Victor has noted, a moral panic is one kind of a mass delusion and it refers to:

A social condition in which a great many people in a society over-react to a newly perceived threat to their well-being from social deviants, even though the actual

that the problem of FMS has been moving through the identified stages of a craze or moral panic.[3] The first stage is characterized by the perception of a threat by a few people who try to spread awareness to the public. In the next phase, the spread of the perceived threat explodes and many people join in the concern. As time goes on, an increasing number of people become skeptical about the threat and consider that it was exaggerated. As resistance spreads, there may be social controversy. Finally, the concern diminishes until it is maintained only by marginal groups. In the case of FMS, the accusations may be waning because this craze has reached a downward phase; or perhaps people have become immune because of the media's deluge of information regarding the controversy.

Another possible interpretation of this data could be that therapists are now being much more cautious and are no longer advising their patients to confront their parents with accusations. Given the guidelines from professional organizations, it is likely that many therapists have reconsidered their past practices.

It is also possible that we see this downward pattern because of the efforts of professionals, who have been effective in educating the public about the problem. People who are accused now do not need to give up their anonymity and can contact the Foundation to get information. Perhaps all of the above are contributing factors to this change.

Data from a 1993 survey of 550 FMS Foundation families showed that in 51% of the families, the fathers were the only ones accused and in 6.5% the mothers were accused. At the same time, 36% of the mothers were accused of active participation with their spouse in the abuse.[4] This means that 42% of mothers are accused of abuse such as inserting umbrella handles or Barbie dolls into the vaginas of infants while changing their diapers. Most remaining mothers were accused of "emotional neglect" and of "not protecting" the accuser. It is difficult to reconcile the high percentage of mothers accused of active sexual abuse of their daughters with the evidence that women rarely abuse very young children and especially female children.[5]

An unusual aspect of the reports to the Foundation is that very few siblings are mentioned as the accused. Research data in a recent article by Levitt and Pinnell reported that sibling incest is far more prevalent than father-daughter incest, with a ratio of 13 to 1.[6] The reverse ratio is reflected in the FMS Foundation data. Fathers were accused of abuse five times more often than siblings were accused. The data is even stranger when it comes to lawsuits. Less than 4% of the repressed memory legal cases that the Foundation has been tracking are being brought only against siblings.

There are virtually no minorities found in the affected families who have contacted the Foundation. The Family Survey[7] data indicate that approximately 30% of the fathers have education beyond college and 28.2 % have completed a four-year college program. Given the fact that the accused are mostly in the 50- through 80-year-old range, this seems a high educational attainment.

That the sample of accused families is so biased—that so many mothers are accused, that so many fathers but not brothers are accused, that the accusations occured over such a short time span—all these data raise many questions.

The presence of retractors provides strong evidence that the recovered memory phenomenon is a moral panic. The fact that some people who had made accusations have come to retract them and, in many cases, have won lawsuits against their former therapists for malpractice is cause for reflection about the FMS phenomenon.

The FMS Foundation January 1997 Survey[8] showed:

7% of families now have a retractor.
25% of accusers have returned without a retraction.

Although the percentage of families who have had a child retract is low, when viewed from a starting point of zero, it represents a significant change. Other factors lead us to believe that many more retractions will follow. Of those people who did retract, more than half initially came back to the families as "returners." Returners are people who return to the family but who do not discuss the accusations. Since 25% of the families now have returners, the pattern will likely continue if we are indeed dealing with a social influence problem. The number of retractors will probably increase. From interviews with families and retractors, we have learned that the process of moving from accuser to retractor frequently takes as many as three years once the process has started.

The comments on some surveys indicated that a few families are cautious and will not accept their child until there is a full apology and retraction. "She has tried, but I have made her unwelcome" or "She tried to, but I wouldn't allow it," are samples of the reactions from those families. Many more families said that they felt that their children were making moves to return but they didn't want to say "yes" because they were not certain. "No, I don't feel that my son has returned, only that the door is not closed as tightly as it was before." Some comments indicated that families had learned to live with the problem. "I still love her and miss her and still hurt a lot—that never seems to go away although the pain is now bearable."[9]

The following comments from those families who reported retractions were interesting:

Daughter ran out of insurance money.

My youngest daughter accused me in 1991 of sexually abusing her after I spent over $200,000 for treatment. After 5 years of hell, my daughter retracted.

It's all like a bad dream now. To be allowed to hold my grandchildren close to me and take them on outings, have them sleep over—the feeling is incredible! I count my blessings.[10]

Why Would They Believe?

Families, professionals and even retractors ask: "How can someone believe in something that is not true, especially when it is horrible and involves people who have been trusted and loved, one's own parents?"

Since belief in recovered repressed memories is held by some but not by others, it seems logical that an individual's suggestibility must play some role. Probably of greater significance, however, is the fact that virtually all of the individuals who developed false memories were vulnerable. People generally go to a therapist when they are down and having difficulty coping. More than 92% of the accusers in the FMS Foundation survey, for example, were distressed enough to turn to an expert for help. They actively sought a person who would give them suggestions about what to do in order to feel better. They were looking for suggestions even before they entered the therapist's office.

Vulnerable people didn't just suddenly spring into being in the late 1980s; they have always been with us but they have not always accused others for their problems.

Satanic ritual abuse expert Jeffrey Victor argues that to understand the rash of false accusations, we must ask about the underlying social conditions that contributed to the credibility of such bizarre stories.

Any adequate explanation cannot be founded upon personality traits, such as superstition, scientific ignorance, suggestibility, or maliciousness. Collective behavior is a product of social dynamics and not a product of personality traits. The popular explanation of attributing moral panics to "contagious hysteria"—meaning a form of temporary, collective psychopathology— simply trivializes these conditions as anomalies. The hysteria explanation ignores the fact that moral panics are quite "normal" (recurrent) events in social systems.[11]

Indeed, as long ago as 1852, Charles Mackay wrote in the preface to *Extraordinary Popular Delusions and the Madness of Crowds*, that whole communities can:

Suddenly fix their minds upon one object,

FRANK & ERNEST® by Bob Thaves

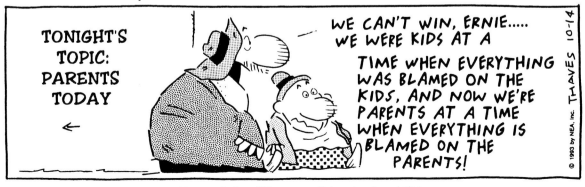

TONIGHT'S TOPIC: PARENTS TODAY ←

WE CAN'T WIN, ERNIE..... WE WERE KIDS AT A TIME WHEN EVERYTHING WAS BLAMED ON THE KIDS, AND NOW WE'RE PARENTS AT A TIME WHEN EVERYTHING IS BLAMED ON THE PARENTS!

THAVES 10-14

© 1993 by NEA, Inc.

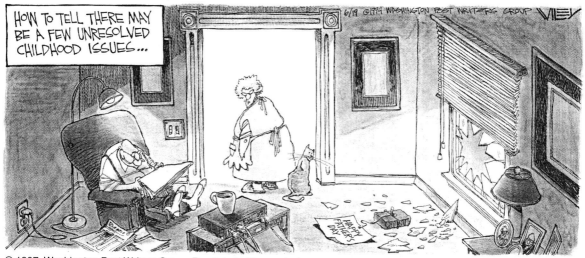

HOW TO TELL THERE MAY BE A FEW UNRESOLVED CHILDHOOD ISSUES...

and go mad in its pursuit; that millions of people become simultaneously impressed with one delusion, and run after it, till their attention is caught by some new folly more captivating than the first.[12]

Collective behavior that somehow goes astray is not something new. History is filled with examples such as the Witch Hunts, the Holocaust and the McCarthy Communism era. Sociologists have come to better understand collective delusions and view some of them as "moral panics."

According to Robert Bartholomew, moral panics are:

Primarily symbolic and rumor-driven, consisting of fear over the exaggerated erosion of traditional values. These moral panics are characterized by self-fulfilling stereotypes of ethnic minorities and deviants who are wrongfully indicted for evil deeds.[13]

The recovered memory movement or the FMS phenomenon begins to make sense when it is seen in the perspective of a moral panic. By the time a cartoonist depicts an issue, it is fairly well understood by the general public. There must be a general consensus of understanding before a cartoon is amusing.

But placing the recovered memory movement within the context of social contagion or moral panic still doesn't explain how someone can come to believe in something that is unbelievable. What does it take?

Authorities and Social Consensus

In a paper presented at the Fourth Annual Convention of the American Psychological Society in June 1992, Robyn M. Dawes, professor of psychology at Carnegie Mellon University, responded to the question of why people believe the unbelievable. In his paper, entitled "Why Believe That for Which There Is No Good Evidence?" Dawes states:

112

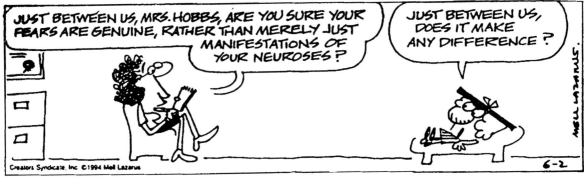

Many people believe in the existence of widespread 'repressed' child sexual abuse and organized satanic cults. Such beliefs occur despite lack of evidence supporting them, influenced instead by reliance on authorities and social consensus. [14]

In the last twenty years, a body of literature has developed, written by self-proclaimed authorities, that defends the theories of repressed memories of childhood abuse. A wide social consensus of psychotherapists, members of the recovery movement, feminists, adherents of various aspects of New Age therapy, talk show hosts and some celebrities developed around these theories.

The recovered memory movement has the two components that Dawes says are necessary for people to believe that for which there is no good evidence: A group of authorities on repressed memories of widespread childhood sexual abuse and a social consensus that has developed with broad support for the theories of these authorities.

We accept authority or we couldn't

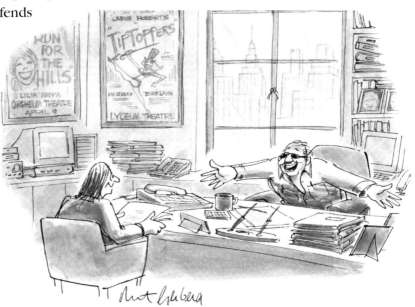

" 'Incest: The Musical'! I love it!"

Drawing by Mort Gerberg; © 1997 The New Yorker Magazine, Inc.

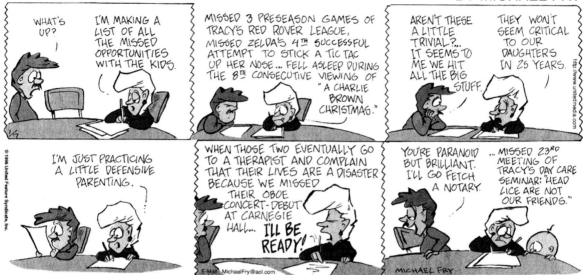

WHAT'S UP?

I'M MAKING A LIST OF ALL THE MISSED OPPORTUNITIES WITH THE KIDS.

MISSED 3 PRESEASON GAMES OF TRACY'S RED ROVER LEAGUE, MISSED ZELDA'S 4TH SUCCESSFUL ATTEMPT TO STICK A TIC TAC UP HER NOSE... FELL ASLEEP DURING THE 8TH CONSECUTIVE VIEWING OF "A CHARLIE BROWN CHRISTMAS."

AREN'T THESE A LITTLE TRIVIAL?... IT SEEMS TO ME WE HIT ALL THE BIG STUFF.

THEY WON'T SEEM CRITICAL TO OUR DAUGHTERS IN 25 YEARS.

I'M JUST PRACTICING A LITTLE DEFENSIVE PARENTING.

WHEN THOSE TWO EVENTUALLY GO TO A THERAPIST AND COMPLAIN THAT THEIR LIVES ARE A DISASTER BECAUSE WE MISSED THEIR OBOE CONCERT-DEBUT AT CARNEGIE HALL... **I'LL BE READY!**

YOU'RE PARANOID BUT BRILLIANT. I'LL GO FETCH A NOTARY.

... MISSED 23RD MEETING OF TRACY'S DAY CARE SEMINAR: "HEAD LICE ARE NOT OUR FRIENDS."

E-Mail: MichaelFry@aol.com   MICHAEL FRY

function in society. If we didn't trust our parents, teachers, doctors, pharmacists, car repair person or the pilot of the plane, we would suffer an inability to function. Dawes claims: "The completely open mind that questions all authority would reside in a body that is a blithering mess."[15]

Good students must trust authority in order to succeed in an educational setting. If they challenged everything presented to them in textbooks and lectures they would never succeed. They must trust that authorities are responsible. Many of the accusers are graduates of some of the finest universities, such as Harvard, Yale, Princeton and Cornell, and they are often successful professionals—nurses, doctors, lawyers, psychotherapists and musicians. The very qualities that made these people excellent students may have made them willing patients in a therapy that provides an apparent learning atmosphere consisting of

books, seminars, therapists and groups. They are provided with book lists and a

BIZARRO   By DAN PIRARO

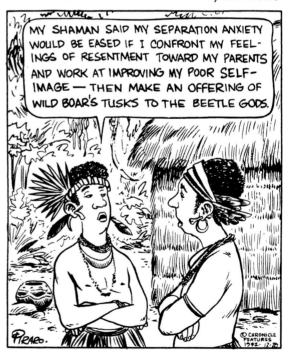

MY SHAMAN SAID MY SEPARATION ANXIETY WOULD BE EASED IF I CONFRONT MY FEELINGS OF RESENTMENT TOWARD MY PARENTS AND WORK AT IMPROVING MY POOR SELF-IMAGE — THEN MAKE AN OFFERING OF WILD BOAR'S TUSKS TO THE BEETLE GODS.

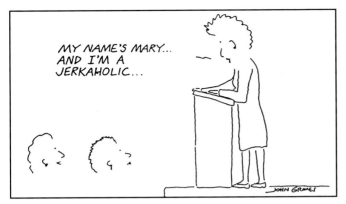

Reprinted courtesy of John Grimes.

structured format of workbooks prescribed by authorities to reach the stated objective of "healing."

Given the circumstances—of intelligent adults seeking answers to problems, authorities who write books and hold training seminars, therapists who guide the process and groups who provide support—is it any wonder that many adult children believe what they are taught to believe? They are taught that millions of adult children have been molested, that any number of ailments are symptoms of the molestation, and that memories have been repressed and can be retrieved in therapy. Therapists and groups then validate the memories.

Once one starts on a course of recovered memory therapy, it becomes a closed system. In 20 years, the ideas formulated by a few therapists permeated our culture and repressed memory therapy was well entrenched. An answer is provided for everything in this type of therapy, as parents and other family members, who try to break through the stone wall that separates them from their accusing children, well know. Anyone who questions the memories is considered to be "in denial"—a euphemism for lying, guilt, evil or stupidity.[16]

Viewed in the historical perspective of social panics, the fact that people can come to believe in something for which there is no evidence is not so strange at all. Often, when "experts" foster a particular position on human behavior, the majority of people unsuspectingly accept the conclusions. This is particularly true when people are vulnerable and turn to the "experts" for advice.

When a closed system that protects a

SALLY FORTH

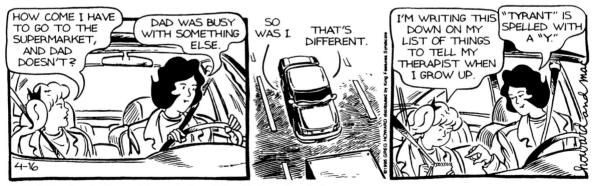

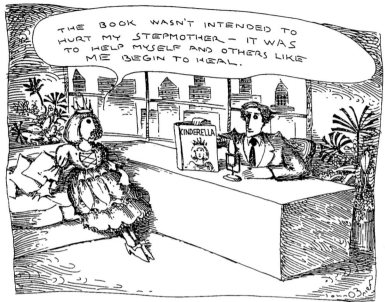

Drawing by John O'Brien; © 1991 The New Yorker Magazine, Inc.

particular belief is breached, however, people move on and slowly abandon the belief. In the case of the recovered memory movement, when memory researchers began to provide scientific facts about the nature of memory, an opening emerged in the closed system. Through scientific information in books, articles, television documentaries and lawsuits, the opening has widened. Slowly, adult children are beginning to relinquish their "recovered memories" and return to the reality of their lives as they were before they entered therapy.

As Charles Mackay noted in 1852: "Men, it has been well said, think in herds; it will be seen that they go mad in herds, while they only recover their senses slowly, and one by one."[17] But it does happen.

Mallard Fillmore

BY BRUCE TINSLEY

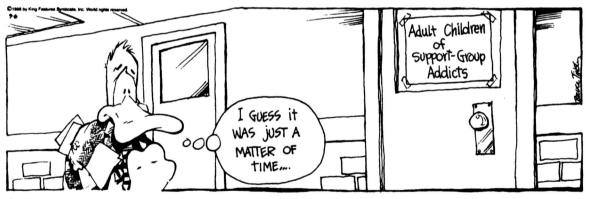

©1996. Reprinted with special permission of King Features Syndicate.

Reference Notes

Introduction

1 Bass, E., & Davis, L. (1988). *The Courage to Heal: A Guide for Women Survivors of Child Sexual Abuse.* New York, NY: Harper & Row, Publishers, 22.

Chapter 1: 100% Dysfunctional

1 Bradshaw, J. (1996). *Bradshaw On: The Family—A New Way of Creating Solid Self-Esteem* (Rev. ed.). Deerfield Beach, FL: Health Communications, Inc.

2 Carl Sagan: A Slayer of Demons. (1996, January/February). *Psychology Today,* 30-65.

3 Blau, M. (1990, July/August). Adult Children Tied to the Past. *<American Health Magazine>*, pp. 55-56. (From <Mental Health 1990> [SIRS Researcher CD-ROM Fall 1996, Art. No. 36]. Boca Raton, FL: SIRS, Inc. [Producer and Distributor].)

Chapter 2: Self-Esteem Overdose

1 Steinem, G. (1992). *Revolution from Within: A Book of Self-Esteem.* Boston, MA: Little, Brown and Company, 67.

2 Ibid., 67.

3 Ibid., 29.

4 Garchik, L. (1996, July 11) Self-esteem overdose dangerous, experts say. *The San Francisco Chronicle.* In *The Palm Beach Post,* p. 5D.

Chapter 3: I'm a Victim, You're a Victim

1 Dineen, T. (1996). *Manufacturing Victims: What the Psychology Industry is doing to People.* Montreal: Robert Davies Publishing, 18.

2 Kaminer, W. (1992). *I'm Dysfunctional, You're Dysfunctional: The Recovery Movement and Other Self-Help Fashions.* Reading, MA: Addison-Wesley Publishing Company, Inc.

3 Ibid., 154.

Chapter 4: From Sinner to Patient to Criminal to Victim

1 Bufe, C. (1991). *Alcoholics Anonymous: Cult or Cure?* San Francisco, CA: See Sharp Press, 19.

2 Ibid., 19-20.

3 Ibid., 36.

4 Ibid., 38.

5 Ibid., 16.

6 Ibid., 41-42.

7 Ibid., 45.

8 Ibid., 47.

9 Ibid., 52.

10 Kaminer, W. (1992). *I'm Dysfunctional, You're Dysfunctional: The Recovery Movement and Other Self-Help Fashions.* Reading, MA: Addison-Wesley Publishing Company, Inc.

Chapter 6: Memory Madness

1 Schacter, D.L., Norman, K.A., & Koutstaal, W. (1997). The recovered memories debate: a cognitive neuroscience perspective. In M.A. Conway, *Recovered Memories and False Memories.* Oxford: Oxford University Press, 63.

2 Bartlett, F.C. (1932). *Remembering: A study in experimental Social Psychology.* Cambridge: Cambridge University Press.

3 Penfield, W. (1975). *The Mystery of the Mind.* Princeton, NJ: Princeton University Press.

4 Loftus, E.F., & Ketcham, K. (1991). *Witness for the Defense: The Accused, the Eye Witness, and the Expert Who Puts Memory on Trial.* New York, NY: St. Martin's Press, 7.

5 Squire, L. (1994, December). Presentation at "Memory and Reality" Conference. Conference co-sponsored by Johns Hopkins Medical Institutions and the False Memory Syndrome Foundation: Baltimore, MD.

6 Neisser, U., & Harsch, N. (1992). Phantom flashbulbs: False recollections of Hearing the News about the *Challenger.* In E. Winograd & U. Neisser (Eds.), *Affect and Accuracy in Recall: Studies of Flashbulb Memories.* (pp. 9-31). New York, NY: Cambridge University Press.

Chapter 7: Under Hypnosis

1 Yapko, M.D. (1994). *Suggestions of Abuse: True and False Memories of Childhood Sexual Trauma.* New York, NY: Simon & Schuster, 57.

2 Ibid., 56.

3 Council on Scientific Affairs. (1985, April 5). Scientific Status of Refreshing Recollection by the Use of Hypnosis. *Journal of the American Medical Association, 253(13),* 1918-1923.

4 Southwick, S.M., Morgan, C.A., Nicolaou, A.L., &

Charney, D.S. (1997, February). Consistency of Memory for Combat-Related Traumatic Events in Veterans of Operation Desert Storm. *American Journal of Psychiatry, 154(2)*.

5 Council on Scientific Affairs. (1985, April 5). Scientific Status of Refreshing Recollection, 1919.

6 Perry, C. (1995). The False Memory Syndrome (FMS) and "Disguised" Hypnosis. *Hypnos, XXII(4)*, 189-197.

7 Poole, D.A., Lindsay, D.S., Memon, A., & Bull, R. (1995). Psychotherapy and the Recovery of Memories of Childhood Sexual Abuse: U.S. and British Practitioners' Opinions, Practices, and Experiences. *Journal of Counseling and Clinical Psychology, 63(3)*, 426-437.

8 Council on Scientific Affairs. (1985, April 5). Scientific Status of Refreshing Recollection, 1918.

9 American Medical Association House of Delegates. (1994). *Report of the Council on Scientific Affairs* (CSA Report 5-A-94). Yank D. Coble, 1.

Chapter 8: Recovering Memories or Myths?

1 Spence, D. (1982). *Narrative Truth and Historical Truth*. New York, NY: W.W. Norton.

2 Pope, H.G. (1997). *Psychology Astray: Fallacies in Studies of "Repressed Memory" and Childhood Trauma*. Boca Raton, FL: Upton Books, 10.

3 Ibid., 11.

4 Ibid., 12.

5 Ibid., 13.

6 Torrey, E.F. (1992). *Freudian Fraud: The Malignant Effect of Freud's Theory on American Thought and Culture*. New York, NY: Harper Collins, 3.

7 Ibid., 5.

8 Pope, H.G. (1997). *Psychology Astray*, 14.

9 Holmes, D.S. (1990). The Evidence for Repression: An Examination of Sixty Years of Research. In J.L. Singer (Ed.). *Repression and Dissociation: Implications for Personality Theory, Psychopathology, and Health*. Chicago, IL: University of Chicago Press, 85.

10 Singer, J.L. (Ed.). (1990). *Repression and Dissociation: Implications for Personality Theory, Psychopathology, and Health*. Chicago, IL: University of Chicago Press, 481.

11 Ibid., 481.

12 Schacter, D.L. (1996). *Searching for Memory: the Brain, the Mind, and the Past*. New York, NY: Basic Books, 262.

13 Phillips, S. (1995, November 8). Innocence Lost: Investigation of Alleged Child Sex Ring. In *Dateline NBC*. New York, NY: National Broadcasting Company, Inc.

Chapter 9: Power of Suggestion

1 Schooler, J.W., Bendiksen, M., & Ambadar, Z. (1997). Taking the middle line: can we accommodate both fabricated and recovered memories of sexual abuse? In M. Conway, *Recovered Memories and False Memories*. Oxford: Oxford University Press, 258.

2 Ibid., 258.

3 Conway, M.A. (1997). *Recovered Memories and False Memories*. Oxford: Oxford University Press, 1.

4 Fivush, R., Pipe, M.E., Murachver, T., & Reese, E. (1997). Events spoken and unspoken: implications of language and memory development for the recovered memory debate. In M.A. Conway, *Recovered Memories and False Memories*. Oxford: Oxford University Press, 30.

5 Ibid., 30.

6 Garry, M., Manning, C.G., & Loftus, E.F. (1996). Imagination Inflation: Imagining a Childhood Event Inflates Confidence that it Occurred. *Psychonomic Bulletin & Review, 3*, 208-214.

7 Roediger, H.L., McDermott, K.B., & Goff, L.M. (1997). Recovery of true and false memories: paradoxical effects of repeating testing. In M.A. Conway, *Recovered Memories and False Memories*. Oxford: Oxford University Press, 133.

8 Asch, S.E. (1952). *Social Psychology*. Englewood Cliffs, NJ: Prentice-Hall.

9 Schooler, J.W. et al., Taking the middle line, 256.

10 Ibid.

Chapter 10: Therapy Gone Crazy

1 Singer, M.T., & Lalich, J. (1996). *"Crazy" Therapies: What Are They? Do They Work?* San Francisco, CA: Jossey-Bass Publishers, 27-28.

2 Ibid., 28.

3 Mack, J.E. (1994). *Abduction: human encounters with aliens*. New York, NY: Scribners.

4 McNamara, E. (1994). *Breakdown: Sex, Suicide, and the Harvard Psychiatrist.* New York, NY: Pocket Books.

5 Council on Scientific Affairs. (1985, April 5). Scientific Status of Refreshing Recollection by the Use of Hypnosis. *Journal of the American Medical Association, 253(13),* 1918-1923.

6 Nash, M. (1987). What, if Anything, is Regressed About Hypnotic Age Regression? A Review of the Empirical Literature. *Psychological Bulletin, 102(1),* 42-52.

7 Ibid., 52.

Chapter 11: The Inner Child

1 Fife, S. (1994, March). Self-Help for New Age Addicts. <*Toronto Life*>, pp. 37-39. (From <Mental Health 1994> [SIRS Researcher CD-ROM Winter 1996, Art. No. 125]. Boca Raton, FL: SIRS, Inc. [Producer and Distributor].)

2 *The Books and Works of Dr. Woititz.* (1996, October 24). [On-line]. Adult Children of Alcoholics. http://www.intac.com/~woy/drwoititz/books.htm#Online Resources

3 From the Adult Children Educational Foundation Computer Bulletin Board. From the Text of *Resources for Adult Children*, a booklet published by Onion House. (1996, October 24). [On-line]. http://www.recovery.org/acoa/whois.acoa.html

4 Katz, S.J., & Liu, A.E. (1991). *The Codependency Conspiracy: How to Break the Recovery Habit and Take Charge of Your Life.* New York, NY: Warner Books, 22.

5 From the Adult Children Educational Foundation Computer Bulletin Board. (See Note #3).

6 Baker, L. (1996, October 23). The Rescue of the Inner Child. [On-line]. http://www.hollys.com/alchemy/rescue.htm

7 Kritsberg, W., & Miller-Kritsberg, C. (1993). *The Invisible Wound: A New Approach to Healing Childhood Sexual Abuse.* New York, NY: Bantam Books, 105.

Chapter 12: A Salesman for the Inner Child

1 Bradshaw, J. (1996). *Bradshaw On: The Family— A New Way of Creating Solid Self-Esteem* (Rev. ed.). Deerfield Beach, FL: Health Communications, Inc.

2 Ibid., 21.

3 Ibid., 94-95.

4 Goldstein, E., & Farmer, K. (1992). *Confabulations: Creating False Memories—Destroying Families.* Boca Raton, FL: SIRS, Inc, 267.

5 Chernoff, G.J. (1990, May/June). John Bradshaw. *Changes For and About Adult Children*, 27-71.

6 Ibid., 70.

7 Ibid., 71.

Chapter 13: In Denial

1 Treatment That's Like 'A Salem Witch Trial'. (1995, November 5). *Mail On Sunday,* p. 39.

2 Personal Communication. (1993, June 24). FMS Family Meeting.

3 *How it Works: Big Book Selections—12 Steps.* (1996, December 19). [On-line]. http://members.aol.com/powerless/HOW.htm#4

4 *How it Works: Big Book Selections—Spiritual Experience.* (1996, December 19). [On-line]. http://members.aol.com/powerless/HOW.htm#4

5 Pendergrast, M. (1995). *Victims of Memory: Sex Abuse Accusations and Shattered Lives.* Hinesburg, VT: Upper Access, Inc.

6 Fife, S. (1994, March). Self-Help for New Age Addicts. <*Toronto Life*>, pp. 37-39. (From <Mental Health 1994> [SIRS Researcher CD-ROM Winter 1996, Art. No. 125]. Boca Raton, FL: SIRS, Inc. [Producer and Distributor].)

7 Tyroler, P.M. (1995, Spring). The Recovered Memory Movement: A Female Perspective. <*Issues in Child Abuse Accusations*>, pp. 72-78. (From <Mental Health 1996> [SIRS Researcher CD-ROM Winter 1996, Art. No. 129]. Boca Raton, FL: SIRS, Inc. [Producer and Distributor].)

8 Bass, E., & Davis, L. (1988). *The Courage to Heal: A Guide for Women Survivors of Child Sexual Abuse.* New York, NY: Harper & Row, Publishers, 87.

9 Pendergrast, M. (1995). *Victims of Memory,* 483.

10 Ibid.

11 Yapko, M.D. (1993). The Seductions of Memory, 34.

12 Ibid.

13 Fredrickson, R. (1992, August). In *Talk of the Nation.* Washington, D.C.: NPR Radio.

14 Yapko, M.D. (1993). The Seductions of Memory, 34.

Chapter 14: Good Parents Are Bad for You

1 FMS Foundation. (1993). *False Memory Syndrome Foundation Family Survey*. Philadelphia, PA.

Chapter 15: Creating Families of Choice, Abandoning Families of Origin

1 Personal Communications. (1996, January 1). *FMS Foundation Newsletter, 5*.

2 Shorter, E. (1997). *A History of Psychiatry: From the Era of the Asylum to the Age of Prozac*. New York, NY: John Wiley & Sons, Inc., 13.

3 Ibid., 131.

4 Mansmann, P.A., & Neuhausel, P.A. (1993, October). Detachment: Applying a well-known concept to ACOA issues. *Professional Counselor*.

5 Ibid.

6 Engel, B. (1989). *The Right to Innocence: Healing the Trauma of Childhood Sexual Abuse*. New York, NY: Ivy Books, 161.

7 Ibid., 166.

8 Briere, J. (1989). *Therapy for Adults Molested as Children: Beyond Survival*. New York, NY: Springer Publishing Co., 142.

9 Courtois, C.A. (1988). *Healing the Incest Wound: Adult Survivors in Therapy*. New York, NY: W.W. Norton & Company.

10 Bass, E., & Davis, L. (1988). *The Courage to Heal: A Guide for Women Survivors of Child Sexual Abuse*. New York, NY: Harper & Row, Publishers, 139.

11 Fredrickson, R. (1992). *Repressed Memories: A Journey to Recovery from Sexual Abuse*. New York, NY: Simon & Schuster, 204.

12 Blackshaw, S., Chandarana, P., Garneau, Y., Merskey, H., & Moscarello, R. (1996). Adult Recovered Memories of Childhood Sexual Abuse. *Canadian Journal of Psychiatry, 41(5)*.

Chapter 16: Post-traumatic Stress Disorder

1 American Psychiatric Association. (1987). *Diagnostic and statistical manual of mental disorders* (3rd ed.). Washington, D.C., 250.

2 Brown, L.S. (1991, Spring). Not outside the range: One feminist perspective on psychic trauma. *American-Imago, 48(1)*, 119-133.

3 Hudson D. (1991, January 17). Too Scared To Remember. In *The Oprah Winfrey Show*. Chicago, IL: Harpo Productions.

4 Suit Against Abusive Therapists Settled. (1995, June 1). *FMS Foundation Newsletter, 4(6)*, 12.

5 Stone, A.A. (1993). Post-Traumatic Stress Disorder and the Law: Critical Review of the New Frontier. *Bulletin of the American Academy of Psychiatry Law, 21(1)*, 23-36.

6 Friedman, M.J. (1996, April). PTSD Diagnosis and Treatment for Mental Health Clinicians. *Community Mental Health Journal, 32(2)*, 173-189.

7 Stone, A.A. (1993). Post-Traumatic Stress Disorder and the Law, 24.

8 Ibid., 25.

9 Pearlman, L.A., & Saakvitne, K. (1995, Summer). *Vicarious Traumatization* [Film]. (Available from Calvacade Productions, 7360 Potter Valley Rd., Ukiah, CA 95482).

10 Ibid.

11 Giller, E. (1995, Spring). How Do Children Cope? The Effect of Dissociative Identity Disorder (Multiple Personality Disorder) On Children of Trauma Survivors. *The Connection, II(2)*, 1-11.

12 Dineen, T. (1996). *Manufacturing Victims: What the Psychology Industry is doing to People*. Montreal: Robert Davies Publishing.

13 Lautens, T. (1996, April 13). Grieving is a growth business for our times. *Globe and Mail*, p. A25.

Chapter 17: Seventy-Six Personalities?

1 Piper, A. (1997). *Hoax & Reality: The Bizarre World of Multiple Personality Disorder*. Northvale, NJ: Jason Aronson Inc., 92.

2 McHugh, P.R. (1995, February). Witches, multiple personalities, and other psychiatric artifacts. *Nature Medicine, 1(2)*, 110-114.

3 Perry, C. (1995). The False Memory Syndrome (FMS) and "Disguised" Hypnosis. *Hypnos, XXII(4)*, 189-197.

4 Kessler, G. (1993, November 28). Mining Gold In Memory Business. *Newsday*, p. 55.

5 Piper, A. (1997). *Hoax & Reality*, xii.

6 Ibid., 20.

7 Ibid., 28.

8 Coons, P.M. (1996, October 28). *Child Abuse And Multiple Personality Disorder*. [On-line]. http://wchat.on.ca/web/asarc/mpd.html

9 Wickens, B. (1989, November 27). Multiple Per-

sonalities: Some Victims Develop A Separate Reality. <*Maclean's*>, pp. 60-61. (From <Mental Health 1989> [SIRS Researcher CD-ROM Fall 1996, Art. No. 14]. Boca Raton, FL: SIRS, Inc. [Producer and Distributor].)

10 Coons, P.M. (1996, October 28). *Child Abuse And Multiple Personality Disorder.* (See Note #8).

11 Kluft, R.P. (1988, December). The Phenomenology and Treatment of Extremely Complex Multiple Personality Disorder. *Dissociation, 1(4),* 47-58.

12 Borch-Jacobsen, M. (1997, April 24). Sybil—The Making of a Disease: An Interview with Dr. Herbert Spiegel. *New York Review of Books,* 60-64.

13 Heaton, J.A., & Wilson, N.L. (1995). *Tuning in Trouble: Talk TV's Destructive Impact on Mental Health.* San Francisco, CA: Jossey-Bass Publishers, 134.

14 Piper, A. (1997, March). A New Day Dawning? *FMS Foundation Newsletter, 6(3),* 8-9.

15 Hipp, D. (1995, November 30-December 6). Rare everywhere but here, MPD is being called an "American disease." *PitchWeekly,* 10-16.

16 Bishop, B. (1997, February 27). Accused blames mental disorder. *The Register-Guard,* pp. 1A, 8A.

17 McBride, J. (1995, November 28). Judge told woman's child self was thief. *Milwaukee Journal Sentinel,* p. 3B.

18 Turkus, J.A. (1996, October 28). *The Spectrum of Dissociative Disorders: An Overview of Diagnosis and Treatment.* [On-line]. http://www.voiceofwomen.com/centerarticle.html

19 Piper, A. (1997). *Hoax & Reality,* 25.

20 Jones, M. (1997, February 4). Doctor accused of bogus therapy, bills. *Milwaukee Journal Sentinel,* pp. 1A, 14A.

Chapter 18: Talk Show Mania

1 Heaton, J.A., & Wilson, N.L. (1995). *Tuning in Trouble: Talk TV's Destructive Impact on Mental Health.* San Francisco, CA: Jossey-Bass Publishers, 1.

2 Ibid,. 2.

3 Goldstein, E., & Farmer, K. (1993). *True Stories of False Memories.* Boca Raton: SIRS Books, 210.

4 Ibid., 211.

5 Ibid., 210.

6 Heaton, J.A. and Wilson, N.L. (1995). *Tuning in Trouble,* 134.

7 Ibid., 134.

8 Bikel, O. (1995, April 4). Divided Memories, Part I—The Hunt for Memory. In *Frontline.* Boston, MA: WGBH Educational Foundation.

Chapter 19: Doing the Work

1 Joseph, N. (1996, November/December). Interview with Charles Whitfield. *The Chorus, VIII(6),* 4-5.

2 Lew, M. (1988). *Victims No Longer: Men Recovering from Incest and Other Sexual Child Abuse.* New York, NY: Harper & Row, Publishers, 141.

3 Personal Communication with Pamela Freyd.

4 *How it Works: Big Book Selections—12 Steps.* (1996, December 19). [On-line]. http://members.aol.com/powerless/HOW.htm#4

5 Remembering Incest & Child Abuse is the First Step to Healing. (1992, July). [Advertisement]. *United Airlines Magazine.*

6 ASCA Co-Dependency Centers. (1991, August/September). [Advertisement]. *Focus.*

7 Baldwin, M. (1988). *Beyond Victim.* Moore Haven, FL: Rainbow Books, 185.

8 Engel, B. (1994). *Families in Recovery: Working Together to Heal the Damage of Childhood Sexual Abuse.* Los Angeles, CA: Lowell House, 25.

9 Blume, E.S. (1990). *Secret Survivors: Uncovering Incest and Its Aftereffects in Women.* New York, NY: Ballantine Books, 274.

10 Lew, M. (1988). *Victims No Longer.* 300-302.

11 Ibid., 211.

12 Ibid., 155.

13 Ibid., 155.

14 Nathan, D. (1992, October). Cry Incest. *Playboy,* 4-164.

15 Ibid., 88.

16 Frankel, F.H. (1994, October). The Concept of Flashbacks in Historical Perspective. *The International Journal of Clinical and Experimental Hypnosis, XLII (4),* 321-335.

17 Maltz, W. (1991). *The Sexual Healing Journey: A Guide for Survivors of Sexual Abuse.* New York, NY: Harper Perennial, 50.

18 Garry, M., Manning, C.G., & Loftus, E.F. (1996).

Imagination Inflation: Imagining a Childhood Event Inflates Confidence that it Occurred. *Psychonomic Bulletin & Review, 3,* 208-214.

19 Briere, J. (1989). *Therapy for Adults Molested as Children: Beyond Survival.* New York, NY: Springer Publishing Company, 101.

Chapter 20: Angry Feminists

1 Goldstein, E., & Farmer, K. (1992). *Confabulations: Creating False Memories–Destroying Families.* Boca Raton, FL: SIRS Books, 308.

2 Ibid., 308-309.

3 Ibid., 309.

4 Ibid.

5 Ibid., 309-310.

6 Steinem, G. (1992). *Revolution from Within: A Book of Self-Esteem.* Boston, MA: Little, Brown and Company, 157.

7 Ibid., 157.

8 Goldstein, E., & Farmer, K. (1992). *Confabulations,* 313.

Chapter 21: Satanic Ritual Abuse

1 Hoover, E. (1997, April 13). Misplaced Memories. *The Sunday Oregonian,* pp. A12-A18.

2 Goldstein, E., & Farmer, K. (1992). *Confabulations: Creating False Memories–Destroying Families.* Boca Raton, FL: SIRS Books, 319.

3 Davis, L. (1991). *Allies in Healing: When the Person You Love Was Sexually Abused as a Child.* New York, NY: Harper Perennial, 132.

4 Bikel, O. (1995, October 24). The Search for Satan. In *Frontline.* Boston, MA: WGBH Educational Foundation.

5 Ross, A.S. (1994, June). Blame It on the Devil. *<Redbook>,* pp. 86+. (From <Family 1994> [SIRS Researcher CD-ROM Fall 1996, Art. No. 33]. Boca Raton, FL: SIRS, Inc. [Producer & Distributor].)

6 Woman Wins $10 M in False Memory Suit. (1997, November 4). *United Press International.*

7 Ross, A.S. (1994, June). Blame It on the Devil. *<Redbook>,* pp. 86+. (See Note #5).

8 Nathan, D., & Snedeker, M. (1995). *Satan's Silence: Ritual Abuse and the Making of a Modern American Witch Hunt.* New York, NY: Basic Books, 107.

9 Ibid., 89.

10 *FBI Study of Childhood Ritual Abuse.* (1996, November 19). [On-line]. http:/web.canlink.com/ocrt/ra_rep03.htm

11 Goleman, D. (1994, October 31). Proof Lacking for Ritual Abuse by Satanists. *The New York Times,* p. A13.

12 Victor, J.S. (1995, January). The Dangers of Moral Panics: What Skeptics (and Everyone Else) Need to Know. *Skeptic, 3(3),* 44-51.

13 Freyd, P. (1996, May 1). Dear Friends, "Does recovered memory therapy help patients get better?" *FMS Foundation Newsletter, 5 (5),* 1.

14 Victims Compensation Administrative Rule Amendments. State of Washington. WAC 296-31-020 Definitions. (1996, December 31).

Chapter 22: Big Business: Self-Help

1 Wills-Brandon, C. (1995). *Another Baby Boomer Phenomenon Bites The Dust: Whatever Happened To The Self Help Movement?* Unpublished Paper.

2 Ibid., 2.

3 Ibid.

4 Kaminer, W. (1992). *I'm Dysfunctional, You're Dysfunctional: The Recovery Movement and Other Self-Help Fashions.* Reading, MA: Addison-Wesley Publishing Company, Inc.

5 Ibid., 165.

Chapter 23: Money Motive

1 Johnston, M. (1997). *Spectral Evidence, The Ramona Case: Incest, Memory, and Truth on Trial in the Napa Valley.* Boston, MA: Houghton Mifflin Company, 77.

2 Dineen, T. (1996). *Manufacturing Victims: What the Psychology Industry is doing to People.* Montreal: Robert Davies Publishing, 197.

3 Sharkey, J. (1994). *Bedlam: Greed, Profiteering, and Fraud in a Mental Health System Gone Crazy.* New York, NY: St. Martin's Press, 142.

4 Rafinski, K. (1996, December 21). Psychiatric hospitals accused of fraud. *The Herald,* pp.1A, 21A.

5 Mulligan, T.S. (1994, April 10). Diet Clinic Tactics Draw Fire. *Los Angeles Times,* pp. A1, A24.

6 Freudenheim, M. (1994, April 12). Corporate-

Paid Psychotherapy: At What Price? *The New York Times,* pp. A1, D2.

7 Sharkey, J. (1994). *Bedlam,* 271.

8 Ibid., 272.

9 Tedford, D. (1994, December 13). Suit hits satanism memories. *Houston Chronicle,* pp.17A, 21A.

10 Tedford, D. (1995, March 8). Woman sues therapists over 500 personalities claim. *Houston Chronicle,* p. 24A.

11 Bikel, O. (1995, October 24). The Search for Satan. In *Frontline.* Boston, MA: WGBH Educational Foundation.

Chapter 24: Insurance Pays

1 Piper, A. (1994, Summer). Treatment of Multiple Personality Disorder: At What Cost? *American Journal of Psychotherapy, 48(3),* 392-400.

2 Ibid., 397.

3 Piper, A. (1997). *Hoax & Reality: The Bizarre World of Multiple Personality Disorder.* Northvale, NJ: Jason Aronson Inc., 152.

4 Bass, E., & Davis, L. (1988). *The Courage to Heal: A Guide for Women Survivors of Child Sexual Abuse.* New York, NY: Harper & Row, Publishers, 311.

5 Grinfeld, M.J. (1996, August). Crime Victims Program Probes Repressed Memory Claims. *Psychiatric Times,* 37-38.

6 Schachner, M. (1994, June 27). 'False Memory' risk surfaces: Providing mental health benefits could lead to lawsuit. *Business Insurance,* 14.

7 Schachner, M. (1994, June 27). 'False Memory' risk surfaces: Providing mental health benefits could lead to lawsuit. *Business Insurance,* 14.

8 Repressed Memory Claims Expected to Soar. (1993, May/June). *The National Psychologist, 4(3).*

9 Ibid.

10 Mental Health Practitioners Application. (1996, January 15). *Rockport Insurance Associates.* Rockport, TX.

11 Davis, R. (1996, November 14). $1 million awarded to settle lawsuit: A State Farm payout ends the suit against a local Assembly of God. *Springfield News-Leader.*

12 2nd patient wins against psychiatrist: Accusation of planting memories brings multimillion-dollar verdict. (1996, January 25). *St. Paul Pioneer Press,* pp. 1B, 4B.

13 Smith, M (1997, August 16). Jury Awards $5.8 Million in Satanic Memories Case. *Houston Chronicle,* p. A1.

14 Woman Wins $10 M in False Memory Suit. (1997, November 4). *United Press International.*

Chapter 25: The Law Steps In

1 Personal Communication. (Letter to False Memory Syndrome Foundation).

2 Alexander, D. (1991, September/October). Still giving the devil more than his due. *The Humanist, 51(5),* 22-42.

3 Bass, E., & Davis, L. (1988). *The Courage to Heal: A Guide for Women Survivors of Child Sexual Abuse.* New York, NY: Harper & Row, Publishers.

4 Ibid., 128.

5 Pendergrast, M. (1995). *Victims of Memory: Sex Abuse Accusations and Shattered Lives.* Hinesburg, VT: Upper Access, Inc., 97-98.

6 Holdings, R. (1997, July1). Repressed Memory Case Suit Man Cleared of Murder Charge Sues Accusers. *The San Francisco Chronicle,* p. A13.

7 NOW Legal Defense and Education Fund. (1992, March). *Legal Remedies For Adult Survivors Of Incest And Child Sexual Abuse* (Rev. ed.). [Legal Resource Kit].

8 Ibid., 1-2.

9 Crnich, J.E., & Crnich, K.A. (1992). *Shifting The Burden of Truth: Suing Child Sexual Abusers—A Legal Guide for Survivors and Their Supporters.* Lake Oswego, OR: Recollex Publishing, 17.

10 Smith, M. (1997, October 29). 5 Psychiatric Workers charged in scam; Insurance allegedly collected after patients linked to ritual abuse. *Houston Chronicle,* p. A1.

11 FMS Foundation Legal Survey. (1997, January).

Conclusion

1 Victor, J.S. (1995, January). The Dangers of Moral Panics: What Skeptics (and Everyone Else) Need to Know. *Skeptic, 3(3),* 44-51.

2 FMS Foundation. (1997, January). *False Memory Syndrome Foundation Family Survey.* Philadelphia, PA.

3 Penrose, L.S. (1952). *Objective Study of Crowd Behavior.* London: H.K. Lewis.

4 FMS Foundation (1993). *False Memory Syndrome Foundation Family Survey.* Philadelphia, PA.

5 Finkelhor, D. (1994, Summer/Fall). Current Information on the Scope and Nature of Child Sexual Abuse. *The Future of Children, 4(2),* 31-53.

6 Levitt, E.E., & Pinnell, C.M. (1995, April). Some Additional Light on the Childhood Sexual Abuse-Psychopathology Axis. *The International Journal of Clinical and Experimental Hypnosis, XLIII(2),* 145-160.

7 FMS Foundation (1993). *False Memory Syndrome Foundation Family Survey.* Philadelphia, PA.

8 FMS Foundation (1997, January). *False Memory Syndrome Foundation Family Survey.* Philadelphia, PA.

9 Ibid.

10 Ibid.

11 Victor, J.S. (1995, January). The Dangers of Moral Panics: What Skeptics (and Everyone Else) Need to Know. *Skeptic, 3(3),* 44-51.

12 Mackay, C. (1980). *Extraordinary Popular Delusions and the Madness of Crowds, Vol. 1.* New York, NY: Harmony Books, xix.

13 Bartholomew, R. (1997, May/June). Collective Delusions: A Skeptic's Guide. *Skeptical Inquirer,* 29-33.

14 Dawes, R.M. (1992, Fall). Why Believe That for Which There Is No Good Evidence? *Issues in Child Abuse Accusations,* 214.

15 Ibid., 215.

16 Goldstein, E., & Farmer, K. (1993). *True Stories of False Memories.* Boca Raton, FL: SIRS Books.

17 Mackay, C. (1980). *Extraordinary Popular Delusions and the Madness of Crowds, XX.*

Bibliography

Alcoholics Anonymous: The Story of How Many Thousands of Men and Women Have Recovered from Alcoholism. (3rd Ed.). (1976). New York, NY: Alcoholics Anonymous World Services, Inc.

American Psychiatric Association. (1987). *Diagnostic and statistical manual of mental disorders* (3rd ed.). Washington D.C.

Asch, S.E. (1952). *Social Psychology.* Englewood Cliffs, NJ: Prentice-Hall.

Baldwin, M. (1988). *Beyond Victim.* Moore Haven, FL: Rainbow Books.

Bartlett, F.C. (1932). *Remembering: A study in experimental Social Psychology.* Cambridge: Cambridge University Press.

Bass, E., & Davis, L. (1988). *The Courage to Heal: A Guide for Women Survivors of Child Sexual Abuse.* New York, NY: Harper & Row, Publishers.

Blume, E.S. (1990). *Secret Survivors: Uncovering Incest and Its Aftereffects in Women.* New York, NY: Ballantine Books.

Bradshaw, J. (1996). *Bradshaw On: The Family—A New Way of Creating Solid Self-Esteem* (Rev. ed.). Deerfield Beach, FL: Health Communications, Inc.

Briere, J. (1989). *Therapy for Adults Molested as Children: Beyond Survival.* New York, NY: Springer Publishing Co.

Bufe, C. (1991). *Alcoholics Anonymous: Cult or Cure?* San Francisco, CA: See Sharp Press.

Canfield, J., & Hansen, M.V. (1993). *Chicken Soup for the Soul: 101 Stories to Open the Heart And Rekindle the Spirit.* Deerfield Beach, FL: Health Communications, Inc.

Conway, M.A. (1997). *Recovered Memories and False Memories.* Oxford: Oxford University Press.

Courtois, C.A. (1988). *Healing the Incest Wound: Adult Survivors in Therapy.* New York, NY: W.W. Norton & Company.

Crnich, J.E., & Crnich, K.A. (1992). *Shifting The Burden of Truth: Suing Child Sexual Abusers—A Legal Guide for Survivors and Their Supporters.* Lake Oswego, OR: Recollex Publishing.

Davis, L. (1991). *Allies in Healing: When the Person You Love Was Sexually Abused as a Child.* New York, NY: Harper Perennial.

Dineen, T. (1996). *Manufacturing Victims: What the Psychology Industry is doing to People.* Montreal: Robert Davies Publishing.

Engel, B. (1989). *The Right to Innocence: Healing the Trauma of Childhood Sexual Abuse.* New York, NY: Ivy Books.

Engel, B. (1994). *Families in Recovery: Working Together to Heal the Damage of Childhood Sexual Abuse.* Los Angeles, CA: Lowell House.

Forward, S., & Buck, C. (1989). *Toxic Parents: Overcoming Their Hurtful Legacy and Reclaiming Your Life.* New York, NY: Bantam Books.

Fredrickson, R. (1992). *Repressed Memories: A Journey to Recovery from Sexual Abuse.* New York, NY: Simon & Schuster.

Goldstein, E., & Farmer, K. (1992). *Confabulations: Creating False Memories—Destroying Families.* Boca Raton, FL: SIRS Books.

Goldstein, E., & Farmer, K. (1993). *True Stories of False Memories.* Boca Raton, FL: SIRS Books.

Heaton, J.A., & Wilson, N.L. (1995). *Tuning in Trouble: Talk TV's Destructive Impact on Mental Health.* San Francisco, CA: Jossey-Bass Publishers.

Johnston, M. (1997). *Spectral Evidence, The Ramona Case: Incest, Memory, and Truth on Trial in the Napa Valley.* Boston, MA: Houghton Mifflin Company.

Kaminer, W. (1992). *I'm Dysfunctional, You're Dysfunctional: The Recovery Movement and Other Self-Help Fashions.* Reading, MA: Addison-Wesley Publishing Company, Inc.

Katz, S.J., & Liu, A.E. (1991). *The Codependency Conspiracy: How to Break the Recovery Habit And Take Charge of Your Life.* New York, NY: Warner Books.

Kritsberg, W., & Miller-Kritsberg, C. (1993). *The Invisible Wound: A New Approach to Healing Childhood Sexual Abuse.* New York, NY: Bantam Books.

Lew, M. (1988). *Victims No Longer: Men Recovering From Incest and Other Sexual Child Abuse.* New York, NY: Harper & Row, Publishers.

Loftus, E.F., & Ketcham, K. (1991). *Witness for the Defense: The Accused, the Eye Witness, and the Expert Who Puts Memory on Trial.* New York, NY: St. Martin's Press.

Mack, J.E. (1994). *Abduction: human encounters with aliens.* New York, NY: Scribners.

Mackay, C. (1980). *Extraordinary Popular Delusions and the Madness of Crowds, Vol. 1.* New York, NY: Harmony Books.

Maltz, W. (1991). *The Sexual Healing Journey: A Guide for Survivors of Sexual Abuse.* New York, NY: Harper Perennial.

McHugh, P.R., & Slavney, P.R. (1986). *The Perspectives of Psychiatry.* Baltimore, MD: The Johns Hopkins University Press.

McNamara, E. (1994). *Breakdown: Sex, Suicide, and the Harvard Psychiatrist.* New York, NY: Pocket Books.

Nathan, D., & Snedeker, M. (1995). *Satan's Silence: Ritual Abuse and the Making of a Modern American Witch Hunt.* New York, NY: Basic Books.

Pendergrast, M. (1995). *Victims of Memory: Sex Abuse Accusations and Shattered Lives.* Hinesburg, VT: Upper Access, Inc.

Penfield, W. (1975). *The Mystery of the Mind.* Princeton, NJ: Princeton University Press.

Piper, A. (1997). *Hoax & Reality: The Bizarre World of Multiple Personality Disorder.* Northvale, NJ: Jason Aronson Inc.

Pope, H.G. (1997). *Psychology Astray: Fallacies in Studies of "Repressed Memory" and Childhood Trauma.* Boca Raton, FL: Upton Books.

Schacter, D.L. (1996). *Searching for Memory: the Brain, the Mind, and the Past.* New York, NY: Basic Books.

Sharkey, J. (1994). *Bedlam: Greed, Profiteering, and Fraud in a Mental Health System Gone Crazy.* New York, NY: St. Martin's Press.

Shorter, E. (1997). *A History of Psychiatry: From the Era of the Asylum to the Age of Prozac.* New York, NY: John Wiley & Sons, Inc.

Singer, J.L. (Ed.). (1990). *Repression and Dissociation: Implications for Personality Theory, Psychopathology, and Health.* Chicago, IL: University of Chicago Press.

Singer, M.T., & Lalich, J. (1996). *"Crazy" Therapies: What Are They? Do They Work?* San Francisco, CA: Jossey-Bass Publishers.

Smith, M., & Pazder, L. (1980). *Michelle Remembers.* New York, NY: Congdon & Lattes.

Spence, D. (1982). *Narrative Truth and Historical Truth.* New York, NY: W.W. Norton.

Steinem, G. (1992). *Revolution from Within: A Book of Self-Esteem.* Boston, MA: Little, Brown and Company.

Thigpen, C.H. and Cleckley, H.M. (1957). *Three Faces of Eve.* New York, NY: McGraw-Hill.

Torrey, E.F. (1992). *Freudian Fraud: The Malignant Effect of Freud's Theory on American Thought and Culture.* New York, NY: Harper Collins.

Wilson, B. (1957). *Alcoholics Anonymous Comes of Age.* New York, NY: Alcoholics Anonymous World Services, Inc.

Winograd, E., & Neisser, U. (Eds.). *Affect and Accu-*

racy in Recall: Studies of Flashbulb Memories. New York, NY: Cambridge University Press.

Woititz, J.G. (1983). *Adult Children Of Alcoholics*. Deerfield Beach, FL: Health Communications, Inc.

Yapko, M.D. (1994). *Suggestions of Abuse: True and False Memories of Chilhood Sexual Trauma*. New York, NY: Simon & Schuster.

FURTHER READINGS

Baker, R. (1992, 1996). *Hidden Memories: Voices and Visions from Within*. Buffalo, NY: Prometheus Books.

Brenneis, C.B. (1997). *Recovered Memories of Trauma: Transferring the Present to the Past*. Madison, CT: International Universities Press, Inc.

Campbell, T. (1994). *Beware the Talking Cure: Psychotherapy May Be Hazardous to Your Health*. Boca Raton, FL: Upton Books.

Ceci, S. & Bruck, M. (1995). *Jeopardy in the Courtroom: A Scientific Analysis of Children's Testimony*. Washington, D.C.: American Psychological Association.

Crews, F. (1995). *The Memory Wars: Freud's Legacy in Dispute*. New York, NY: New York Review of Books.

Dawes, R. (1994). *House of Cards: Psychology and Psychiatry Built on Myth*. New York, NY: Free Press.

Gordon, B. (1995). *Memory: Remembering and Forgetting in Everyday Life*. New York, NY: Mastermedia Limited.

Hacking, I. (1995). *Rewriting the Soul: Multiple Personality and the Sciences of Memory*. Princeton, NJ: Princeton University Press.

Hagen, M. (1997). *Whores of the Court*. New York, NY: Regan Books.

Kotre, J. (1995). *White Gloves: How We Create Ourselves Through Memory*. New York, NY: Free Press.

Laframboise, D. (1996). *Princess at the Window: A New Gender Morality*. Toronto: Penguin.

LeDoux, J. (1996). *The Emotional Brain: The Mysterious Underpinnings of Emotional Life*. New York, NY: Simon & Schuster.

Loftus, E. & Ketcham, K. (1994). *The Myth of Repressed Memory*. New York, NY: St. Martin's Press.

MacLean, H.N. (1993). *Once Upon A Time: A True Story of Memory, Murder, and the Law*. New York, NY: Harper Collins.

Merskey, H. (1995). *Analysis of Hysteria: Understanding Conversion and Dissociation*. UK: Gaskell.

Ofshe, R. & Watters, E. (1994). *Making Monsters: False Memory, Psychotherapy and Sexual Hysteria*. New York, NY: Charles Scribner's Sons.

Richardson, J., Best, J., & Bromley, D. (Eds.). (1991). *The Satanism Scare*. New York, NY: Aldine de Gruyter.

Sagan, C. (1995). *The Demon-Haunted World: Science as a Candle in the Dark*. New York, NY: Random House.

Showalter, E. (1997). *Hystories: Hysterical Epidemics and Modern Media*. New York, NY: Columbia University Press.

Slovenko, R. (1995). *Psychiatry and Criminal Culpability*. New York, NY: Wiley.

Smith, S. (1995). *Survivor Psychology: The Dark Side of a Mental Health Mission*. Boca Raton, FL: Upton Books.

Sommers, C.H. (1994). *Who Stole Feminism: How Women Have Betrayed Women*. New York, NY: Simon & Schuster.

Spanos, N. (1996). *Multiple Personality and False Memory*. Washington, D.C.: American Psychological Association.

Victor, J. (1993). *Satanic Panic: The Creation of a Contemporary Legend*. Chicago, IL: Open Court Publishing.

Wakefield, H. & Underwager, R. (1994). *Return of the Furies: Analysis of Recovery Memory Therapy*. Chicago, IL: Open Court Publishing.

Webster, R. (1995). *Why Freud Was Wrong: Sin, Science and Psychoanalysis*. New York, NY: Basic Books.

Wright, L. (1994). *Remembering Satan: Case of Recovered Memory and the Shattering of an American Family*. New York, NY: Knopf.

Young, A. (1996). *Harmony of Illusions: Invention Post-Traumatic Stress Disorder*. Princeton, NJ: Princeton University Press.

Recommended Professional Reports

American Psychiatric Association. (1993, December 12). *Statement on Memories of Sexual Abuse.* Washington, D.C.

American Psychological Association. (1995, August 10). *Questions and Answers About Memories of Childhood Abuse.* Washington, D.C.

American Psychological Association. (1996). *Working Group on Investigation of Memories of Childhood Abuse: Final Report.* Washington, D.C.: Alpert, J., Brown, L., Ceci, S., Courtois, C., Loftus, E., & Ornstein, P.

American Society of Clinical Hypnosis. (1994). *Clinical Hypnosis and Memory: Guidelines for Clinicians and for Forensic Hypnosis.* Des Plaines, IL: Hypnosis and Memory Committee of ASCH.

Australian Psychological Society Limited, Board of Directors. (1994, October 1). *Guidelines Relating to the Reporting of Recovered Memories.* Melbourne, Australia.

British Psychological Society. (1995, January). *Recovered Memories: The Report of the Working Party of the British Psychological Society.* Leicester, UK: British Psychological Society.

National Association of Social Workers. (1996, June). *Evaluation and Treatment of Adults With the Possibility of Recovered Memories of Childhood Sexual Abuse.* Washington, D.C.: NASW National Council on the Practice of Clinical Social Work.

Recommended Journal Issues

American Journal of Clinical Hypnosis. (1994, January)

Applied Cognitive Psychology. (1994, August).

Canadian Psychiatric Association. (1996, March 25). Position Statement, "Adult Recovered Memories of Childhood Sexual Abuse." *Canadian Journal of Psychiatry, 41(5).*

Consciousness and Cognition. (1994, September-December).

Counseling Psychologist. (1995, April).

International Journal of Clinical and Experimental Hypnosis (Part 1). (1994, October).

Journal of Psychiatry & Law. (1995, Fall).

Journal of Traumatic Stress. (1995, October).

Memory & Language. (1996, April).

Psychiatric Annals. (1995, December).

Psychiatry & Law. (1996, Summer).

Psychanalytic Dialogues, 6(2). (1996).

Psychological Inquiry, 7(2). (1996).

Psychology & Theology. (1992, Fall).

Skeptic. (1995, Fall).

INDEX